UNDER THAT CALAMITY

BY JOHN PERCEVAL

EDITED BY LINDSEY GRUBBS

CLOCKWORK EDITIONS

Carmilla
by Joseph Sheridan LeFanu
edited by Carmen Maria Machado

*Medusa's Daughters: Magic and Monstronsity
from Women Writers of the Fin-de-Siècle*
edited by Theodora Goss

The King in Yellow
by Robert W. Chambers
edited by John Edgar Browning

A NARRATIVE

OF THE

TREATMENT EXPERIENCED

BY A

GENTLEMAN,

DURING A STATE OF

MENTAL DERANGEMENT;

DESIGNED

TO EXPLAIN THE CAUSES AND THE NATURE

OF

INSANITY,

AND TO EXPOSE THE INJUDICIOUS CONDUCT PURSUED
TOWARDS MANY UNFORTUNATE SUFFERERS

UNDER THAT CALAMITY.

by John Perceval

Edited by Lindsey Grubbs

"Infandum Regina jubes renovare dolorem
Quæque ipse miserrima vidi
Et quorum pars magna fui."*

LANTERNFISH PRESS

PHILADELPHIA

---

* Perceval draws this quote from Book II of Virgil's *Aeneid*, deleting a line that references Troy. H. Rushton Fairclough's translation for the Loeb Classical Library reads, "Too deep for words, O queen, is the grief you bid me renew...—the sights most piteous that I saw myself and wherein I played no small role."

UNDER THAT CALAMITY
This text was initially printed anonymously in 1838 as *A narrative of the treatment experienced by a gentleman, during a state of mental derangement; designed to explain the causes and the nature of insanity, and to expose the injudicious conduct pursued towards many unfortunate sufferers under that Calamity.*

Lanternfish Press
21 S 11th St. Office #404
Philadelphia, PA 19107

lanternfishpress.com

INTRODUCTION AND NOTES: © 2022 Lindsey Grubbs

ARCHIVAL SUPPORT: Rachel D'Agostino, Curator of Printed Books for the Library Company of Philadelphia.

COVER ART: Scientific illustration by Camillo Golgi, 1903. Digital image courtesy of OHSU Historical Collections & Archives in Portland, Oregon.

COVER DESIGN: Kimberly Glyder

ILLUSTRATIONS: Digital images courtesy of the Library Company of Philadelphia and the Wellcome Collection.

Printed in the United States of America
Library of Congress Control Number: 2021944809
Print ISBN: 978-1-941360-63-7
Digital ISBN: 978-1-941360-64-4

26 25 24 23 22   1 2 3 4 5

Dedicated to the Alleged Lunatics' Friend
Society and those who followed.

CONTENTS

INTRODUCTION

In July 1859, John Perceval appeared before Parliament's Select Committee on Lunatics—a group appointed to investigate the state of English laws regulating the treatment of those deemed mad.[1] The hearing had been spurred by one of the century's "lunacy panics," a rise in public sentiments of suspicion towards alienists (medical specialists in insanity). This suspicion was occasioned by the enormous power granted to physicians: by law, any person could be confined to an asylum if the person recommending it submitted two certificates from physicians who had separately examined the patient.[2] In 1859, a series of highly publicized cases pressed the government to act.

The year prior, the writer Rosina Bulwer Lytton had expressed her loathing of her husband, the politician and author Edward Bulwer-Lytton, during an acrimonious separation. After she crashed a campaign event to rail against his election, she was abducted and placed in an asylum. Her release was secured in part through public outcry against the misdiagnosis of her anger as insanity, and against a system that allowed a wife to be put out of the way so simply. In another, Mary Jane Turner was incarcerated by a doctor who admitted to verbally abusing and isolating her. She eventually escaped by throwing knotted bedsheets out the window. Cases of women confined by their husbands and families seemed particularly successful in raising alarm, and in both Britain and the United States, highly publicized cases of wrongful confinement sparked anxiety about the use of medical power to deprive sane persons of their liberty. Still, the hearings were dominated by male speakers like Perceval.

Addressing the Select Committee as a reformer, Perceval declared himself "the attorney-general of all Her Majesty's madmen."[3] He had earned this self-appointed title through decades of advocacy: as a founding member of the delightfully named Alleged Lunatics' Friend Society (ALFS), Perceval had fought against wrongful confinement and the mistreatment of the mad. The organization lobbied governmental leaders, defended "alleged lunatics" in court, and agitated for reform through print, working for almost fifteen years to bring about a hearing like the one where Perceval now spoke. Like many other members of the ALFS, Perceval became involved in the cause through personal experience. During a period of religious delusion in 1830, his family had placed him in Brislington House, an elite "reformed" asylum run by the Fox family near Bristol— an experience he records at length in the volume you hold in your hands, which documents both his symptoms and his mistreatment.[4] After thirteen months of treatment (or, as he would put it, *despite* thirteen months of treatment), Perceval recovered. However, he was not given his liberty but was instead transferred to Dr. Newington's asylum at Ticehurst. With no effective avenues to pursue his freedom, and with those around him prejudiced against his sanity, he remained confined against his will for two more years.[5] Outraged by his treatment, Perceval would use print, pen, and voice in pursuit of an England more hospitable for the eccentric and the mad.

Born in 1803, John Perceval was one of Prime Minister Spencer Perceval and Jane Wilson's thirteen children.[6] When John was nine, his father was assassinated by a merchant with a grudge against the government. He would go on to complete his primary education at the elite Harrow School and receive an army commission through family connections, serving without combat in Portugal and Ireland. He ultimately found this earthly work incompatible with his strong religious sentiments and, at the age of twenty-seven, sold his commission to attend Oxford. This move would be short-lived: along with his eldest brother, Spencer, he left for Row, Scotland, to investigate reports of miracles occurring amid a religious sect led by Edward Irving. John and Spencer were excited by rumors of faith healing and speaking in tongues—evidence of God's continued action in the world. After hearing those speaking in tongues firsthand, John found himself similarly inspired. (In his second memoir, he would note that the Irvingites had disavowed him and claimed that his voices were prompted by a devil, not God.) He attributed the onset of his religious delusions to this exciting atmosphere.[7]

After leaving Row in a state of agitation, Perceval traveled to Dublin, where he was devastated by his own hypocrisy when he employed a sex worker. After he contracted syphilis from the encounter, he was tormented by intrusive thoughts pitting his doctor's advice against a divine voice rejecting it. His behavior became increasingly erratic, and in December of 1830 he was restrained at an inn. After a period of isolation and restraint—to which he attributed his further decline—Spencer took John to Brislington House, where he remained until May of 1832. This asylum was among the most expensive in the nation, and his family supposedly spent three hundred guineas (roughly $30,000 today) for fourteen months of treatment.[8]

Brislington House was established at the beginning of the nineteenth century by Edward Long Fox, a Quaker physician ascribing to new philosophies.[9] Before the nineteenth century, the mad tended to be cared for (or, very often, abused) in their own homes or in public institutions like poorhouses. While asylums existed—the infamous "Bedlam" was founded in the thirteenth century as the Priory of St. Mary of Bethlehem, though it would not become an institution for the insane until a later date— these institutions were relatively small and usually housed the poor temporarily. Among the upper classes, troubled or troublesome family members were often sent to private "madhouses," sometimes more genteelly labeled "nervous clinics," which offered containment rather than cure. In the early nineteenth century, though, the care of the insane solidified into a medical specialty, and adherents began to develop faith in the curative possibilities of confinement. In a time of increasing professionalization and specialization, the new class of asylum physicians claimed to reject earlier "medical" treatments for insanity, like bleeding, purging, and manacles. Instead, they relied on "moral treatment" ("moral" meaning something more like "psychological" than "ethical"). They believed the asylum could provide structure, recreation, labor, kindness, and doctor-patient relationships that would coach the mad back to sanity as they learned "self-restraint" in an attempt to please their keepers.

By the time of Perceval's incarceration in the early 1830s, the asylum was run not by the elder Dr. Fox, who remained on the premises, but his sons, Francis and Charles. In a pamphlet published a few years after Perceval's stay, the younger Doctors Fox described the grounds of the asylum and their treatment principles.[10] They begin the advertisement on the defensive, noting their awareness that "great abuses have formerly existed in houses devoted to care of the insane and that the public mind has been prejudiced against the whole system of lunatic asylums, by the detail of some cases of ignorance and cruelty." But many prior abuses, they suggest, were owing to organizational problems: the mingling of sexes and classes, of violent and convalescent patients, or of curable and incurable ones. The Foxes solved such problems architecturally. Male and female quarters were entirely separated (a situation about which Perceval complained routinely). Even the weekly Church of England services, performed in the laundry, were structured such that, while both men and women could see the minister, they could not see one another. (Segregated, too, were faiths—Catholics, Unitarians, and Quakers were forbidden to attend these services without the express desire of the family.)

In the male and female wings, patients were further divided into three classes. These classes never mingled, to prevent envy and to protect "persons of rank and quality from an indiscriminate association with those of inferior manners and condition, which otherwise on their mutual recovery might lead to inconvenient, if not detrimental acquaintance." (In a letter later published by Perceval, we learn that exceptions were made for men of middle ranks who excelled enough in sport to entertain the upper classes.) Each class had two sitting rooms, which further divided the patients into violent and convalescent cases. The property also had separate housing for those who had physical ailments needing care or quarantine, as well as private quarters for the especially wealthy, "some of which," the Foxes bragged, "are at present inhabited by members of the nobility."

The Doctors Fox claimed to reject intimidation, corporal punishment, and personal restraint for the management of the insane. They note that, when transitioning from private care to the asylum, "all personal coercion is suspended," and patients were nursed to health through cultivating "habits of the greatest simplicity and regularity." They rejected medical interventions, like bleeding, noting that their own philosophy saw the body as a system. Thus, they encouraged frequent exercise, extolling the virtues of their bowling greens, cricket fields, greyhound parties, and indoor games. They remarked on patients' easy access to outdoor spaces—mounded in such a way that inmates could take in views of the secluded wooded estate and its surroundings despite the walls built to prevent escape.

I have described the Foxes' philosophy at length because, as the reader of this volume will see, their representation is at odds with Perceval's. (Perceval refused even to call Brislington House an "asylum," preferring the pejorative "mad-house," as he thought the association of the word asylum with peace made its use here a "cruel mockery and revolting duplicity.") He wrote his narrative a few years after his release from Ticehurst, the second madhouse. By then he had married Anna Gardiner, a cheesemonger's daughter, and relocated to Paris, where in 1835 he wrote his recollections. In 1838, against his family's wishes, he anonymously published the first edition of his memoir, which you hold. In it, he describes the nature of his insanity and the cruelty of the treatment he received. He describes traumatic bleedings, unwilling dunkings in the cold bath, lack of exercise, and extensive time in straitjackets and manacles, which the asylum claimed to use sparingly. Perceval's narrative makes plain two things: first, that even "enlightened" practitioners relied more on the older methods than they advertised. He concludes that "the greatest part of the violence that occurs in lunatic asyla, is to be attributed to the conduct of those who are dealing with the disease, not to the disease itself." Second, that the newer, gentler techniques came with their own problems, namely the surveillance and infantilization of patients. In Perceval's words, "they addressed me as a child, and I did not understand them, because I knew I was a man." Where alienists saw a system of "soothing," Perceval saw "repression by mildness and coaxing" that left discharged patients to a "milk sop existence."[11] Indeed, "the very acts of impatience and impetuosity" that signaled to Perceval that he was returning to his "sound senses" and responding to his environment appropriately were "held up by my doctor to the keepers as the signs of mania; the very disorder for which I was to be detained." Thus, while Perceval was in the asylum at an optimistic time for the profession—a time when cure through incarceration seemed possible, and before asylums became brutal warehouses for the mad[12]—his own recollections show that the faith in medical progress recorded by asylum physicians was not felt by all.

At the end of his first account, Perceval describes leaving Brislington for a new asylum. The final page of the book leaves a tantalizing hint: "Note.—The Letters promised in an appendix at the end of the volume have been suppressed on the ground of delicacy by the advice of my Publisher." These letters, though, did not remain suppressed for long. Two years later, Perceval followed up with a second volume that bore the same name but was more sequel than revision. After four chapters of review, Perceval charges forward to provide an account of his second incarceration. Having had his identity revealed by a Scottish magazine editor, his new title page bore the name of John Perceval, Esq. This book boasted 430 pages to the first's 278 and included a blistering 28-page preface. He writes of physicians as "despots" and "mean-minded upstart adventurers" and describes being consigned to keepers as passing into the "lowest and coarsest, to the profanest, and most *criminal* hands." The Lunacy Commissioners, meant to safeguard the rights of those incarcerated, are themselves "more criminal than the lunatic doctors." Abandoned by those meant to protect him, he lays out three goals for writing: to reform the laws of commitment, to reform the management of the asylum, and to reform the way families handle the care of their lunatic members.

In pursuit of those goals, Perceval composed an eclectic volume, which at times resembles a printed scrapbook more than a clear narrative: he weaves together anti-asylum polemic; copies of letters written to and from the asylum; excerpts from his daily asylum journal ("Wednesday, May 2.—Serenaded this morning by the seraphine;—at half-past one, a wrestling match;—about three, fiddling and more wrestling. This an asylum for nervous patients!"); poems by Byron edited to include lines more applicable to his own plight; and, at one point, a script of dialogue that occurred following an escape attempt, with his and Dr. Newington's roles rendered as "Mr. N." and "*Lunatic!*" On the 430th and final page of the text, the narrative remains unresolved, spanning only the first few months of his two-year commitment in Ticehurt. He concludes abruptly: "But more of this anon, if my countrymen will allow me to continue my narrative."

The second volume makes even more plain several points articulated in the first, and so I relate them here for the benefit of the reader. With his identity revealed, Perceval lays out his frustration with his family, whom he does not suspect of devious motives but finds weak-willed and lacking common sense in their continuous accession to his doctors' wishes. His legal complaints against Dr. Fox are clarified, too, as he outlines the charges he hopes to file, revolving most seriously around the forced use of cold baths in the winter—which he believes damaged his health—but also around failures of hygiene and grooming.

If the first volume focused largely on the mistreatment of the lunatic, the second turns more fully to the fate of the *alleged* lunatic. At the end of his time at Dr. Fox's madhouse and the beginning of his time at Dr. Newington's, Perceval believed he had been returned to sanity. Though noting the lingering physical and mental effects of both his lunacy and his incarceration, and even the continuance of voices that he had learned how to ignore, he is entirely clear: at this point, he was able to make decisions on his own behalf, and his decision was to leave. Notably, he did not even request complete freedom but instead a more discreet and quiet location, like a family home, in which to recover. As his published letters show, Perceval made a clear and convincing case. Importantly, he notes that perfect sanity is not required to justify autonomy. On his ride from Brislington to Ticehurst, he finds himself often unable to speak, sings to himself in tongues, and continues to experience strong religious sentiments. Yet, he writes, "altho' I could not call myself of sound mind, I had no disposition to do injury to myself or others."

At Ticehurst, though, he would discover the difficulty facing the recovered lunatic: all his actions were interpreted as pathology. Perceval had grown a long beard and hair as a rebellion against the dehumanizing system of grooming employed in Dr. Fox's asylum, where his prized whiskers were shaved and his hair cut into a species of mullet. But for Newington, the visiting physicians, and the commissioners meant to safeguard Perceval's rights, this style was evidence of continued insanity. Even more problematically, his anger at the family who refused to listen to him and at the physician who had abused him was rendered not righteous fury but lunatic mania when read through the lens of an assumed diagnosis. In describing the options available for redress, he asks, "How was a man confessing himself to have been a lunatic, mistrusted doubtless, in some degree, even by those who knew him best, to obtain credence?"

While the second volume shows Perceval gaining clarity on the injustices that would fuel a lifetime of advocacy, it also reveals more strongly the absolute snobbishness justifying many of his positions. While the asylum at Brislington was segregated by class, its highest class was not high enough for Perceval, since it included anyone who could pay for the honor. In a letter, he talks about the trials of confinement with twelve other patients: "individuals, for the most part, of no rank, no birth, little education, no manners, and thoroughly dead to all gentlemanly and moral feelings, and I may say moral habits, to which I have been accustomed, to which I have been educated, and to which I have clung from my father's cradle until now." He bristles at Dr. Newington reading and controlling his mail not only because of the inherent intrusion into his privacy but because of his disgust at such an upstart acting as "the keeper of my conscience": "These are like swine or sloths set to judge over the manners of greyhounds and fleet coursers." As he claims in the preface, "The revolutionary and infidel liberal principles of the present day mock at high birth, and insolently sneer at long descent as a mere accident—a matter of chance, endowing men with no distinction. Let a lunatic teach them—for the author learnt to feel it when lunatic—that there is no such thing as chance—no such thing as accident."

Perceval's memoirs would receive mixed reviews, including those that criticized his classism. But excerpts circulated through papers, as in the case of *Littell's Spirit of the Magazines and Annuals*, which itself pulled the text from *Tait's Magazine*. This passage appeared as "Reminiscences of a Religious Maniac" after the preface of Charles Dickens' *Nicholas Nickleby*.[13] Despite this traffic in the press, though, Perceval's text failed to raise the kind of alarm occasioned by some other accounts of incarceration.

While Perceval's memoir alone did not much advance the needle of reform, he fortuitously found his way to a group of like-minded individuals. The same year that Perceval published his narrative, Richard Paternoster was released from a forty-one-day involuntary commitment to Kensington

House Asylum following a financial dispute with his father. His abduction was witnessed by reporters, which, along with the energetic advocacy of his landlady, helped lend press attention to the case. His case was tried by the Metropolitan Commissioners, who voted 6-4 for his release. He alleged abuse and even murder in the asylum and advertised his experience widely. Perceval reached out to him, as did several others, and a group assembled around shared interests. One early member was William Bailey, who had been placed in an asylum by his wife despite several physicians testifying to his sanity and was shuffled between asylums whenever an interview with the Commissioners approached. Perceval and Paternoster lurked under Bailey's window until he threw them documents allowing them to make the case for his sanity and release. A fourth accomplice, Lewis Phillips, had been put away by his brothers until he agreed to give up his stake in their business; they then shipped him overseas. Rounding out the group were Richard Saumarez, who was not himself a patient but had two brothers confined, and John Parkin, an epidemiologist who spent time in an asylum. Thus began the organization that would become the Alleged Lunatics' Friend Society.[14]

They had several goals: they sought jury hearings for all accusations of insanity, because doctors' financial and professional interests made them unreliable witnesses. Similarly, they wanted wealthy lunatics' money to be put into government bonds rather than family hands, reducing the incentives for confinement. For those in asylums, they wanted a clear appeal process and coroners' hearings for suspicious deaths. They applied political pressure, harshly criticizing a system that asked the lunacy commission to regulate and monitor itself. When they heard in 1845 that changes to the lunacy laws were forthcoming, they formalized the society at last, with Perceval serving as honorary secretary. Overall, they professed three major goals: to alter lunacy laws, to assist those discharged from asylums, and to increase public sympathy for the insane.

The 1845 legislation was a disappointment. The bar for certification became modestly higher: both of the evaluations by physicians had to happen within seven days, and the doctors had to provide explanations if they recommended commitment. (Another provision said that all counties must have asylums for paupers—the ALFS, though, seem largely concerned with middle- and upper-class concerns.) Most of the ALFS positions were ignored, for example, that patients should know the nature of their commitment and evidence for it and be allowed to attend meetings on their status. Rejected, too, were voluntary halfway houses, protections for property, and inquests into deaths. But while their legislative attempts often failed, they continued to put pressure on individual politicians—a task that Perceval took to particularly strongly given his family connections.

Beyond legislative reforms, they focused on justice in court cases and the transformation of public opinion on the insane. Often these strands were linked: investigations like an 1852 inquiry into abuses at Bethlem helped increase oversight in the Lunacy Acts of 1853. Of the society's fifty to sixty members, around ten were lawyers, and between 1845 and 1863, they took on more than seventy patients' cases. Some were high-profile wrongful confinement cases, like that of Louisa Nottidge, incarcerated so she wouldn't donate her inheritance to a religious sect. In the case of Anne Nottingham, they went so far as to help her escape.

But despite the "alleged" in their name, they often tried cases not of wrongful confinement but of abuse.

As an advocate, Perceval took up both individual cases of mistreatment and a public campaign for reforms of not only laws but of sentiments. One media campaign Perceval lodged against the Northampton Hospital resulted in new staff and treatment protocols. While the press responded well to the society in some ways, they worked against them in others: they were as likely to publish a sensational tale of crime by a dangerous lunatic as they were a case of wrongful confinement. Perceval worked to disrupt these dominant narratives. He advocated on behalf of Arthur Legent Pearce, incarcerated in Bedlam for criminal insanity following an attack on his wife. To help raise funds for Pearce's care, he edited a volume of the prisoner's poetry, *Poems by a Prisoner in Bethlehem*. Another of Perceval's key successes was the case of Professor Edward Peithman, who had spent fourteen years in an asylum after trying to tell Prince Albert about his views on a national education system. The success of the Peithman case garnered further attention to and cases for the ALFS. Perceval would later report that one asylum keeper greeted him by saying, "I assure you I would rather see the devil in my asylum than you."[15]

Legislatively, though, other than minor progress on provisions like disallowing hearsay evidence on certificates, reform seemed out of reach. Thus, the 1858 lunacy panics presented a prime opportunity for a renewed agenda. Meeting to discuss high-profile cases like Bulwer Lytton's, they petitioned again for a hearing and were finally granted the request. The head of the Select Committee on Lunacy would be Home Secretary Spencer Horatio Walpole— Perceval's brother-in-law.

Perceval's testimony at these meetings tackled two problems: on the first day, he focused on recommendations to eliminate wrongful confinements. On the second, he spoke to improving the conditions in asylums. He criticized both the lack of stronger laws and the failures of the Commissioners to uphold existing ones. Many of his arguments at the Select Committee emerged directly from his experience. He argued especially vehemently against the existence of private asylums for the wealthy, like the ones where he had been kept, because he believed the high fees created too much of an incentive to claim that a perfectly sane, or at least harmlessly mad, patient needed confinement. (He was not advocating for equality of treatment here but rather for the creation of facilities suitable for the upper classes in public asylums.) He argued against the institutionalization of the founders of new religions, noting that Christ and his apostles were themselves accused of madness, and castigates those who are quick to judge as mad "any man who is a little original."

He argued for voluntary asylums and halfway houses, for civil involvement in certification and appeal, for the free passage of patients' mail (except in the case of women writing immoral things), for the safeguarding of patients' belongings, for asylum attendants who were "young men of the aristocracy," and for removing families' incentives to incarcerate harmlessly eccentric family members. While he said that the "furiously insane" or "evidently imbecile" should be excepted, the certification process in general should be more arduous. When they ask if this is only for the wealthy, he claimed somewhat unconvincingly: "I do not care about fortunes; I look to a person's civil rights and their personal freedom." To improve the asylums themselves, he calls for better attendants, less reliance on violence, and sin-gle-patient houses. He believes clergy visits would help to solve patients' "sort of cold feeling and exile from society." Perceval's wide-ranging testimony was followed by one of the commissioners Perceval had criticized. The man was quick to seize one of Perceval's points upon which they could agree: yes, much of the problem was down to the low-class attendants.

The committee found some of the ALFS positions convincing, though Perceval found their report unsatisfy-ing: they recommended a jury for all cases, not just for the wealthy; that all certificates should be signed by magistrates, as they were for paupers; and that certifications should be renewed every three months. Even these modest recom-mendations, though, were rejected by the Lord Chancellor. Following this defeat, the ALFS began to fade away, ceasing to operate entirely in 1863. Thirteen years later, Perceval would die at the age of seventy-three in the Munster House Asylum. He saw few of his desired reforms in place.[16]

Perceval's legacy, though, did not end there. Though often derided and lacking public support, the Alleged Lunatics' Friends helped shift the conversation about patient rights. Other patient-led organizations would take up the advocacy mantle, most notably the Lunacy Law Reform Association, founded by Louisa Lowe following her own incarceration at Brislington (due in large part to her spiritualist beliefs). Not until 1890 did many of the reforms for which Perceval advocated begin to pass, including the involvement of civil authorities in the commitment process and the replace-ment of indefinite certifications with fixed-term renewable ones. Further, after two visits from a physician, a patient could be *de*certified and removed from the asylum if not a danger to themselves. Ultimately, many of the reforms that had seemed radical at Perceval's time—like the posting of patients' rights in asylums, documentation of dissatisfaction with confinement, transitional housing for those leaving or on their way to asylums, freedom of mail, and improved licensure for nursing staff—would be enacted.[17]

One hundred and twenty-three years after the initial publication of Perceval's account, it found a new audience. The 1960s saw a wave of protest literature rivaling that of the 1850s, as anti-psychiatry and anti-institutional sentiments blossomed across the decade in response to evidence of the oppressive conditions of the hospitalized. In 1948, Albert Deutsch's exposé *The Shame of the States* had revealed the horrifying conditions in public asylums, while the same year, Mary Jane Ward's semi-autobiographical novel *The Snake Pit* was turned into a film starring Olivia de Havilland. The most extreme position was taken by "anti-psychiatrists" who argued the profession was more interested in controlling social deviance than treating illness. Authors like R.D. Laing went so far as to say that psychotic symptoms were battles with social repression, and Thomas Szasz published *The Myth of Mental Illness* in 1960. More typically, critics interrogated the history and logic of institutional care, and Szasz's text was followed by Michel Foucault's *Madness and Civilization* and Irving Goffman's *Asylums*. Many of Goffman's critiques—that asylums were infantilizing and oppressive—will be familiar to readers of Perceval's far earlier text. Members of this movement recovered historical accounts of mistreatment and false confinement. As in the nineteenth-century lunacy panics, accounts by women—like the American Elizabeth Packard, incarcerated for holding different religious principles than her husband—were particularly popular for their ability to demonstrate the ways in which psychiatric power could be deployed to maintain social hierarchy and order.

It was as part of this wave of academic and popular interest in the status of psychiatry that the anthropologist Gregory Bateson published a new edition of Perceval's text as *Perceval's Narrative: A Patient's Account of His Psychosis* in 1961. The work went through multiple printings and brought Perceval into the canon of madness.[18] Perceval was excerpted in Szasz's 1973 compilation of historical texts on involuntary commitment from Daniel Defoe to Sylvia Plath under the title "The Lunatic's Protest." In 1982, an excerpt would appear in *A Mad People's History of Madness*—a collection of first-person writing by people diagnosed with mental illness.[19]

Bateson, known for ethnographic fieldwork in New Guinea and Bali with his first wife Margaret Mead, turned toward the study of schizophrenia in the 1950s. Working with a group of researchers, he developed a theory that the symptoms of schizophrenia arose from communication conflicts within families. It was as part of this work that he reintroduced Perceval's text, which he accordingly read through this lens. Bateson stressed the scientific value of the account, which he writes "makes contributions to our knowledge of schizophrenia." Much of his introduction is spent psychoanalyzing Perceval, concluding that the symptoms of schizophrenia have curative abilities to repair damage to selfhood caused by competing personal traits. He calls psychosis not so much a disease as a "painful initiatory ceremony conducted by the self." In contrast to other memoirs of mental illness, which Bateson suggests are "specimens of psychotic or post-psychotic utterance," Perceval offers "scientific contributions in their own right," making "discoveries" that are useful to "modern psychiatry."[20] The back of the 1974 edition claims that this is an "account of schizophrenia" from the pen of "one certifiably insane." Within the nineteenth-century context of lunacy certification, though, "certifiably insane" was a far more loaded term, pointing less to scientific fact and more to systems of medical power and legal judgment.

The historians Richard Hunter and Ida MacAlpine reviewed Bateson's publication, criticizing his lack of historical context and his editorial overzealousness in combining the two volumes, and they stressed Perceval's role in advocacy on behalf of the mentally ill as the "gad-fly" of the Commissioners in Lunacy. Still, they note that first-person accounts provide access to the "aberrations" of the human mind "in pure culture."[21] Perceval certainly attempts to describe the working of insanity. But this laboratory metaphor, in which text is rendered into Petri dish, reveals that even those paying homage to Perceval's legacy tend to see him as object of study more than expert in his own right.

Undoubtedly, Perceval tells a privileged story of forced commitment. He was in the best hospital that money could buy, and many of his complaints are about lack of decorum rather than outright abuse. Nevertheless, he paints a compelling and convincing portrait of the lack of respect and humility bound up in the care of the lunatic. One particularly important lesson Perceval relates is about the unparalleled expertise of the lunatic on matters of lunacy. He writes: "Having been under the care of four lunatic doctors, whose systems of treatment differ widely from each other—having conversed with two others, and having lived in company with Lunatics, observing their manners, and reflecting on my own, I deem that alone sufficient excuse for setting forth my griefs and theirs, before men of understanding, to whom I desire to be supposed addressing myself."

Perceval takes pains to highlight the hypocrisy of those who claim that lunacy is a great mystery but also claim to know with certainty what is best for patients. He takes particular aim at the use of restraint and forced indolence, and at the blanket pronouncement that interaction with the family is bad for mental health—an argument commonly used at the time to justify the asylum system. He offers his testimony as counterweight: "Feeling the ignorance to be in one sense real, which all of you confess on your lips, listen to one who can instruct you." He entreats his readers to read his text charitably and to take his complaints seriously, not just writing them off as the words of a lunatic: "Bring the ears and the minds of children, children as you are, or pretend to be, in knowledge—not believing without questioning, but questioning that you may believe."

His request for his contemporaries to read with curiosity rather than prejudice serves as a reminder, too, for the modern reader. If Perceval had difficulty getting taken seriously upon regaining his sanity in the asylum, he would face the same problem in his writing. He knows that his critics cast him off as "a madman or a fool."[22] One scholar writing about the progressive and humanistic goals of Dr. Fox and Brislington house suggests that "Perceval's highly coloured account has to be treated with caution," though there may be "an element of truth" in it.[23] The reader is not similarly cautioned, however, when the source is the Foxes' own advertising material. While he ultimately believes Perceval that restraint was used, he takes this fact as evidence that the violence of certain lunatics forced the otherwise enlightened doctors to use harsher methods—not of Perceval's insight on matters of treatment. Such suspicious readings are even more notable given Perceval's habit of admitting to delusion and his frank statements of failed memory.

What, then, did Perceval, expert in lunacy, recommend? He wanted common-sense, rather than medically specialized, treatment. His scorn for mad-doctors ("that race of presuming upstarts" whose "end is to make money, not to make whole") comes across clearly in blistering sarcasm: "His companion seemed so stupid, and so like a man of the world of a common and vague stamp of mind, that I thought it perhaps still more hopeless to address him. ...I have since learned, that this wise second to Dr. P. was a lunatic doctor, celebrated in Dublin. And to that, in part, I cannot help attributing my subsequent misfortunes." Not only were mad-doctors fools, but so were those who bowed to their expertise, and he noted that his case turned for the worse when his physician "submitted me to the treatment of a lunatic doctor," and thus "submitted his own judgment along with it." Particularly galling was his family's reliance on the word of this (lower-than-his-own-class) physician over his own.

Laying out his treatment in plain terms, he demonstrates its absurdity:

> Tie an active limbed, active minded, actively
> imagining young man in bed, hand and foot, for

a fortnight, drench him with medicines, slops,
clysters; when reduced to the extreme of nervous
debility, and his derangement is successfully confirmed, manacle him down for twenty-four hours
in the cabin of a ship; then for a whole year shut
him up from six, A.M. to eight, P.M. regardless
of his former habits, in a room full of strangers,
ranting, noisy, quarrelsome, revolting, madmen;
give him no tonic medicines, no peculiar treatment
or attention, leave him to a nondescript domestic,
now brushing his clothes, sweeping the floors,
serving at table, now his companion out of doors,
now his bed-room companion; now throwing him
on the floor, kneeling on him, striking him under
all these distressing and perplexing circumstances;
debar him from all conversation with his superiors,
all communication with his friends, all insight
into their motives, every impression of sane and
well-behaved society! surprise him on all occasions,
never leave harassing him night or day, or at meals;
whether you bleed him to death, or cut his hair,
show the same utter contempt for his will or inclination; do all in your power to crush every germ of
self-respect that may yet remain, or rise up in his
bosom; manacle him as you would a felon; expose
him to ridicule, and give him no opportunity of
retirement or self-reflection; and what are you to
expect.

More substantial than his critique of his physical treatment was his critique of his mental and moral treatment.
He attributes his cure to times when he was allowed to act

on delusions and see that the consequence was not what he imagined. For example, had his keepers, rather than restraining him, allowed him to look out the window he imagined a scene of horrors beyond, he would have been confronted with his own delusion. Instead, time and again, "I was left a lunatic to my lunatic imagination to supply me with a reason." Early in his delusions, he writes, "Had my brother but said to himself, 'there is something strange here; I will try to understand it'—had he but pretended to give credit to what I said, and reasoned with me on the matter revealed to me, acknowledging the possibility, but denying or questioning the divine nature of my inspirations; I should, perhaps, have been soon rescued from my dreadful situation, and saved from ruin: but it was not so." He demands more addresses to the reason of the patient.

One final lesson emerges from a feature that distinguishes Perceval's text from others of the time. In contrast to sensational tales about perfectly rational people being abducted and placed in asylums for the benefit of their greedy family members—accounts that took their power from the notion that it could happen to anyone—Perceval is entirely forthcoming about his lunacy. Indeed, describing the "causes and nature of insanity" from an insider's view is one of the primary goals of his work. While "wrongful confinement" tales from "alleged lunatics" shored up the notion that there was such a thing as "rightful confinement" for "true lunatics," Perceval's narrative pushes us to ask messier questions. What do we owe the mad? How should we manage those who, as Perceval readily admits, will strike their keepers or attempt to harm themselves as soon as they are freed from restraint? These questions would be echoed in the ALFS's advocacy agenda—while relying on "alleged lunacy" to appeal to societal fears of wrongful confinement, they fought on behalf of both the misdiagnosed and the mistreated.

I don't mean to overstate the progressiveness of the ALFS position. They were not abolitionists. As Perceval would write, the ALFS aimed to improve the system "not in order to throw difficulties in the way of persons who are really insane and dangerous, or who need protection, being restrained."[24] Still, they asserted that the net had been cast far too wide, until it caught harmless eccentrics, convalescents who needed a calmer place to recover, and those who challenged Victorian moral propriety. While attempting to retract the borders of the land of the mad, he asked also for sympathy for those who lived within them.

Ultimately, Perceval emphasizes that the horrors of lunacy did not emerge only from the mind of the deluded patient but also from the society that treated them. People treat the mad "with lunatic cruelty, and the insanest mismanagement." The need for change, he asserts, lies in the system of treatment, not in the lunatic himself. Indeed, he rejects the shame he has been asked to bear: "so weak are so called sane man's imbecilities; imbecilities, such as make me less ashamed of having been a mad-man, when I think of the disgrace of such conduct, of such credulity, lightness, and triviality, unaccompanied and unexcused by disease."

The text of the volume that follows is drawn from Perceval's 1838 edition. Bateson's text combines editions, deleting those chapters he finds "contentious and repetitive." I take a different approach, presenting the first edition largely as published, even where Perceval struggled, in his own words, to "write orderly." The reader will notice that the narrative does not always move chronologically. While he presents his biography in roughly a straight line until he reaches Dr. Fox's doors, his account at that point moves thematically rather than temporally, cycling through time marked by seasons rather than dates and returning to the same season time and again.

I have retained nineteenth-century and British spelling variants and have made no attempt to regularize Perceval's grammar. While his deployment of commas and his use of exclamations and question marks mid-sentence appear unconventional to the modern reader, they provide a sense of his rhythms as a writer and thinker. For example, he writes, "Particularly, finding the tones vary, I asked which is the voice of God? but my suspicions were soon lulled again." In running straight into the "but" without capitalization, he typographically signals the connection between the thoughts, and the intrusiveness of the question. Perceval also combines certain compound words (like rendering "ill-treatment" as "illtreatment") and separates others ("every thing" for "everything"), but these spellings are not unique to Perceval, and on both counts I find his elision or expansion potentially meaningful.

My editorial intrusions are mostly twofold: I have left Perceval's occasional misspellings alone but have corrected obvious typos (i.e., "submittted" for "submitted"), and have silently deleted the spaces that appeared before many forms of punctuation. In these edits, I have made assumptions about which features were introduced by Perceval and which through the printing process, and admit the possibility that I have left misspellings introduced by the printer, or that Perceval was deeply attached to his well-spaced punctuation. Overall, though, I have attempted to remain true to Perceval's text, following his own lead: "My reader, I have had great difficulty to get even thus far, but, if after this you meet with more irregularity and abruptness of style, and change of manner, recollect how painful a task I am engaged in, and pass it over."

NOTES

1   Perceval and his contemporaries wrote of "derangement," "lunacy," "imbecility," and "insanity," and in this introduction I rely on the terms that would have been significant to him rather than applying anachronistic modern language.

2   For more on "lunacy panics," see Peter McCandless, "Liberty and Lunacy: The Victorians and Wrongful Confinement," in *The Social History of Psychiatry in the Victorian Era*, ed. Andrew Scull (Philadelphia: University of Pennsylvania Press, 1981) and Sarah Wise, *Inconvenient People: Lunacy, Liberty, and the Mad-Doctors in Victorian England*, (Berkeley: Counterpoint, 2012). Many of the accounts of wrongful confinement I mention in this introduction are drawn from the latter text.

3   *Report from the Select Committee on Lunatics; Together with the Proceedings of the Committee, Minutes of Evidence, Appendix, and Index*, printed for the House of Commons, 1859, 23.

4   This text was initially printed anonymously as *A narrative of the treatment experienced by a gentleman, during a state of mental derangement; designed to explain the causes and the nature of insanity, and to expose the injudicious conduct pursued towards many unfortunate sufferers under that Calamity* (London: Effingham Wilson, 1838).

5   Perceval would go into greater detail about his experience at Ticehurst in the second, de-anonymized edition of his text, bearing the same name and published in 1840, again by Effingham Wilson.

6   Biographical details are drawn from Perceval's two accounts; the introduction to Gregory Bateson, ed., *Perceval's Narrative: A Patient's Account of His Psychosis, 1830-1832* (New York: William Morrow & Company, 1974); Richard Hunter and Ida Macalpine, "John Thomas Perceval (1803-1876) Patient and Reformer," *Medical History* 6, no. 4 (1962): 391-95; and Wise, *Inconvenient People*.

7   Indeed, religion and spirituality were very commonly a factor in cases of contested sanity, highlighting the difficulty of drawing lines between sanity and insanity. Atheism was certainly grounds for suspecting someone's sanity, but so was claiming to hear the voice of the God that all were meant to believe existed. Certainly, not all evangelicals were considered insane—Spencer would even become one of the twelve Apostles of the Irvingite faith.

8 By way of anachronistic comparison, a two-week stay at McLean Hospital's elite "Pavilion" in the United States costs $59,500 and is not billable to insurance. See "The Pavilion," McLean Hospital, accessed November 19, 2021, https://www.mcleanhospital.org/treatment/pavilion.

9 For an account of Fox's medical philosophy and description of Brislington House, see Leonard Smith, "A Gentleman's Mad-Doctor in Georgian England: Edward Long Fox and Brislington House," *History of Psychiatry* 19, no. 2 (2008): 163-184 and Clare Hickman, "The Picturesque at Brislington House, Bristol: The Role of Landscape in Relation to the Treatment of Mental Illness in the Early Nineteenth-Century Asylum," *Garden History* 33, no. 1 (2005): 47-60. More general information on the history of psychiatry and the asylum is drawn from Edward Shorter, *A History of Psychiatry: From the Era of the Asylum to the Age of Prozac* (New York: Wiley, 1997).

10 This illustrated guide is Francis Fox and Charles Fox, *History and Present State of Brislington House near Bristol, an Asylum for the Cure and Reception of Insane Persons* (Bristol: Light and Ridler, 1836.)

11 Quoted from Nicholas Hervey, "Advocacy or Folly: The Alleged Lunatics' Friend Society, 1845-63," *Medical History* 30 (1986): 245-275.

12 In 1827 the average English asylum had one hundred and sixteen patients. By 1910 it would have one thousand and seventy two. See Shorter, *History of Psychiatry*, 18.

13 "Reminiscences of a Religious Maniac," *Littell's Spirit of the Magazines and Annuals* 3, 1839, 762-775.

14 The following material on the ALFS is drawn from Wise, *Inconvenient People*, Hunter and Macalpine, "John Thomas Perceval," and Nicholas Hervey, "Advocacy or Folly: The Alleged Lunatics' Friend Society, 1845-63," *Medical History* 30 (1986): 245-275.

15 *Report from the Select Committee*, 22.

16 Wise, *Inconvenient People*, 290.

17 Hervey, "Advocacy or Folly."

18 It was reprinted the following year in London by Hogarth Press and yet again in 1974. This introduction quotes the 1974 edition cited above.

19 Thomas Szasz, ed., *The Age of Madness* (Garden City, NY: Anchor Books, 1973) and Dale Peterson, ed., *A Mad People's History of Madness* (University of Pittsburgh Press, 1982).

20   Bateson, *Perceval's Narrative*, xix, v.

21   Hunter and MacAlpine, "John Thomas Perceval," 391.

22   John Perceval, "Treatment of the Insane," *Provincial Medical and Surgical Journal* 15, no. 24 (1851): 665-666.

23   Smith, "A Gentleman's Mad-Doctor," 179 & 173.

24   Perceval, "Treatment of the Insane," 666.

UNDER THAT CALAMITY

CHAPTER I

IN THE YEAR 1830, I was unfortunately deprived of the use of reason. This calamity befel me about Christmas. I was then in Dublin. The Almighty allowed my mind to become a ruin under sickness—delusions of a religious nature, and treatment contrary to nature. My soul survived that ruin. As I was a victim at first, in part to the ignorance or want of thought of my physician, so I was consigned afterwards to the control of other medical men, whose habitual cruelty, and worse than ignorance—*charlatanism*—became the severest part of my most severe scourge. I suffered great cruelties, accompanied with much wrong and insult; first, during my confinement, when in a state of childish imbecility in the year 1831; secondly, during my recovery from that state, between November, 1831, and May, 1832; thirdly, during the remainder of the year 1832, and the year 1833, when I considered myself to be of sane mind. Having been under the care of four lunatic doctors, whose systems of treatment differ widely from each other—having conversed with two others, and having lived in company with Lunatics, observing their manners, and reflecting on

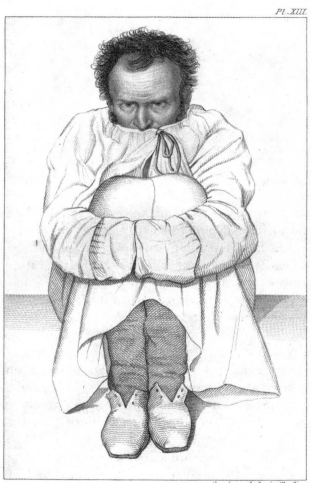

Pl. XIII.

Gravé par Ambroise Tardieu

A patient exhibiting "dementia" from French alienist Étienne
Esquirol's 1838 textbook *Des maladies mentales considérées
sous les rapports médical, hygiénique et médico-légal.*

my own, I deem that alone sufficient excuse for setting forth my griefs and theirs, before men of understanding, to whom I desire to be supposed addressing myself, and for obtruding upon them more of my personal history than might otherwise be prudent or becoming. Because I wish to stir up an intelligent and active sympathy, in behalf of the most wretched, the most oppressed, the only helpless of mankind, by proving with how much needless tyranny they are treated—and this in mockery—by men who pretend indeed their cure, but who are, in reality, their tormentors and destroyers.

I open my mouth for the dumb; and let it be recollected, that I write in defence of youth and old age, of female delicacy, modesty, and tenderness, not only of man and of manhood—surrendered up in weakness to indecent exposure, disgusting outrage, or uncalled for violence—that I write for the few who are objects of suspicion and alarm,—to society, who too much engrossed in business or in pleasure to exercise reflection, are equally capable of treating these objects of their dread and insolence, with lunatic cruelty, and the insanest mismanagement; being deprived, like them, of understanding, by exaggerated and unreasonable fear, but not like them by illness, of the guilt of their misconduct. The subject to which I direct attention, is also one on which, my readers, according to man's wont, the wisest of you are hasty to decide in action, or to hazard an opinion in proportion even to your ignorance.

In the name of humanity, then, in the name of modesty, in the name of wisdom, I intreat you to place yourselves in the position of those whose sufferings I describe, before you attempt to discuss what course is to be pursued towards them. Feel for them; try to defend them. Be their friends,—argue not hostilely. Feeling the ignorance to be in one sense real, which all of you confess on your lips, listen to one who can instruct you. Bring the ears and the minds of children, children as you are, or pretend to be, in knowledge—not believing without questioning, but questioning that you may believe.

CHAPTER II

I WAS BORN of parents powerful, honourable, and happy, till a cruel blow deprived my mother of a husband, and her family of a father. He was a minister of state; and my relations rank among the aristocracy and wealth of my country.[1] I was educated in the bosom of peace and plenty, in principles of delicacy and decorum, in modest and temperate habits, and in the observance of, and real veneration for, the religion of my country.

At the age of seventeen, I left the public school,[2] at which I had passed seven years, not without credit, to study with a private tutor, and the next year, the inclination I had formed in childhood for a military life still predominating, my family procured me a commission in a regiment of cavalry; two

---

1   John Thomas Perceval's father was Spencer Perceval, the Prime Minister of the United Kingdom. The elder Perceval was assassinated in 1812 by John Bellingham, a merchant aggrieved with the government. Many thought Bellingham mad, but he denied it. Perceval was nine when his father was killed. His vagueness about his father's position here serves as a reminder that the first edition of the text was anonymous—though his identity was revealed shortly after publication.

2   In England, a "public school" is a private school. Perceval attended Harrow, an elite boarding school outside of London.

troops of that regiment being shortly after reduced, I was placed on half-pay, and allowed next year to exchange into the Guards. I owed both my commissions to the kindness of the Duke of York, and to the attention of his secretary, Sir Herbert Taylor, who were glad to show their respect for the memory of my father.[3] I had been nursed in the lap of ease, and scrupulous morality; I now entered the school of polite and gentlemanly behaviour.

I passed my life in the Guards quiet and unobserved. I had, as at school, three or four friends, and no very extensive general acquaintance. If I was remarkable in society for any thing, it was for occasional absence of mind, and for my gravity and silence when the levity of my companions transgressed the bounds of decorum, and made light of religion, or offended against morality. I was firm also in resisting all attempts to drive me by ridicule into intemperance. In private I had severe conflict of mind upon the truth and nature of the Christian religion, accompanied with acute agony at my own inconsistency of conduct and sentiment with the principles of duty and feeling taught by Jesus and his apostles; and mingled with astonishment at the whirlpool of dissipation, and contradiction in society around me. After several years inward suffering and perplexity, question and examination, I found at last, for a time, peace, and joy, and triumph, as I imagined, in the doctrines usually styled "evangelical."[4] Till then the sacrifice of Jesus Christ, instead

---

3 At this time, officer commissions in the military could be bought and sold rather than earned through experience. The Duke of York, otherwise known as Prince Frederick, was the second son of King George III—the so-called "Mad King."

4 Evangelical approaches to religion, which encouraged people to read scripture, pray, and pursue salvation through an individual relationship to Christ, grew throughout the nineteenth century through a series of religious

of being a message of gladness, had always been to me one of increasing woe and shame; as a sinner, to whom it made the law more binding, the offences against the law more ungrateful—the heinousness of crime deeper, in proportion to my conception of the boundless love of Almighty God. Then I understood that the law was done away in Christ, and liberty given to the mind, so that the soul might choose gratefully what it could not be driven to by fear. In the year 1829, my conduct first became decided and extreme, through the active principle instilled by the doctrines I have named; and in the spring of the year 1830, influenced chiefly by this new principle of action, I obtained permission to sell my commission in the Guards.

Since, however, many reasons combined to determine this resolution, I will mention them briefly. Not unconscious that they may excite the ridicule of many, nor that a few may accuse me of vanity in the detail, as well as in what I have already written. But my object is, without affecting more candour than is necessary, and without pretending to excuse or to blame, to show in my own instance the kind of disposition that was exposed to treatment of too sad a nature. For in arguing on the treatment of lunatics, mankind usually, though confessing ignorance, set out with the conceit that ill-treatment (or, to use the well-disguised language of the physicians, "wholesome restraint," or "wholesome correction") is necessary; and proceed as if this

---

revivals. In the context of the national religion of the Church of England, evangelicalism likely seemed suspiciously enthusiastic. In both the United States and the United Kingdom, religious beliefs out of the mainstream were commonly cited as evidence of—or fertile ground for—madness, and asylum records from the period are full of cases of "religious mania." Although indicating the influence of religion on his insanity here, Perceval later argued against the institutionalization of the founders of new religions, noting that Jesus and the apostles were themselves called mad.

conceit were a principle established on evidence, instead of wickedly admitted through the very ignorance they avow. Next, in hearing the complaints of lunatics, they are prone to the suspicion, that the evil conduct of the complainant brought both his calamity and his persecutions upon him; and not that mild and civil, and even childlike, as well as childish natures, are submitted to cruel tortures from profane hands—through the supineness of society in abandoning individuals, without knowledge of the disease or discrimination, into the hands of men of little education, and of low origin, implicitly relying on their pretensions, yet as men dealing only practically with such patients.[5]

---

5 While expressing his frustration with a medical culture that blamed patients and claimed expertise unsubstantiated by true knowledge of the workings of the mind, Perceval also makes clear his class biases: as working professionals, physicians were second-class citizens whose authority over his care was particularly galling.

CHAPTER III

IN THE FIRST PLACE, the evangelical opinions I had embraced, containing, as I imagined, the light of everlasting truth, given me freely through the election of God the Father, for the sake of the obedience, and sacrifice of Jesus Christ, and to the end that His own glory might be made manifest, in changing a vile and weak creature into the likeness of Divine holiness, excited in me gratitude and fear: gratitude for the gift given me, and for that election; and fear of the wrath of God, if I disobeyed the end for which it was given. That which had been done for me, I thought it my duty to preach to others, and to explain the doctrines, whereby I had been saved. Moved by these arguments, I spoke and acted in open confession of my faith, a line of conduct not very agreeable to the army, even if called for, and judicious. Being then in Dublin, I attached myself to a society for reading the scriptures to the Irish poor; I attended the regimental schools; I read the service to a detachment I commanded, as the men had not seats provided for them in church;—I tried to establish a reading-room for the soldiers of my battalion;—I procured religious and other books for the sick in hospital, and being afterwards quartered in town, hearing that two battalions of guards and the recruits, through the neglect of the Chaplain and indifference of the commanding officers, had been for a long time upon one pretence or another without opportunity of attending divine service at all, by privately applying to a clergyman in Westminster, and to an officer of one battalion of like sentiments to my own, we procured seats for the men in a large chapel, belonging to the church of England. I had obtained the like permission from a clergyman of the established church for the other battalion, when I found that this conduct excited suspicion and offence. Both Colonel and Chaplains showed some symptoms of chagrin—they charged me with having sent the men to a dissenting minister. My conduct in reading the service to the detachment I for a time commanded near Dublin, in circulating religious books, and in other respects, drew on me also private animadversions, although in no instance did I transgress military discipline; in the first case, I acted only in obedience to the regulations of the army. Now, though not sure that I was doing quite right, I felt inclined to do more;—for I outfaced slander and cavil thus, that even if I were in the extreme, it was but fair that one should be in the extreme in the cause of Christ, when so many were running recklessly a course of gaiety and dissoluteness. But as I really esteemed my superior officer, who was both kind, intelligent, and actively beneficent; and as I loved good discipline, I judged it prudent to withdraw from a scene of constant conflict with my own conscience, where I was tempted to act unwisely, and where I might be led into quarrel with those whom I loved and respected, through conduct I might afterwards sincerely repent of.

In the next place, I was led by a passage in the New Testament, exhorting the Christian to choose *liberty* rather than slavery.[6] I conceived this advice applicable to a situation like my own, where I was so much confined in the liberty of speech and conversation with the private soldier, by the strict discipline of the service. After that, I reflected on my natural disposition, talents, and acquirements. I was fond of quiet, seclusion, and study; unused to boisterous sports, untried in situations requiring promptitude and decision. I had a long time mistrusted my courage, and presence of mind, and had feared, that in the hour of trial, I might do discredit to the regiment and to my own name. In 1827, in Portugal, I had seen a bloodless campaign, excepting the assassination of one or two of the men and outrages upon the officers, unatoned for. Though the scene was novel and the country beautiful, my mind was fatigued by the long marches between the towns—to do nothing. I disliked idleness, accompanied by suspense of mind, separation from all means of regular study, and the absence of the attractions of female society. One night we had encamped, and I came to the resolution that my life might be a very romantic one, but that it was far from being agreeable. I was cheerful and contented, and glad that we had a fine night, but I judged coolly, and with reason, that a better cause than that of kings and constitutions, the instruments after all, and the embodyings of the spirit of Satan, was required to justify the sacrifice of happiness and comfort to one, who needed not to gain his *living* by cutting his neighbour's throat. I felt too, in the end, that we had been made fools and tools of. My tastes,

---

6   Possibly Galatians 5:1: "Stand fast therefore in the liberty wherewith Christ hath made us free, and be not entangled again with the yoke of bondage." Bible verses in footnotes are drawn from the King James Bible.

therefore, were little suited to a military life, and my talents and acquirements not much more. I had already too much religion, to enjoy thoughtless dissipation, and too much reflection, to be the blind instrument of power; though I had been a long time in the army, and had devoted part of that time to acquire an insight into the principles of the profession, and a knowledge of languages, in hopes of being of service to my country; yet my attention had been chiefly absorbed by points of evidence and doctrine connected with religion, and I found myself at last, better adapted to confute a Papist or an infidel, without committing myself, than to manœuvre a battalion, or even to direct a company.

Religion therefore and propriety thus dictating to me, affection also had its weight. My youngest brother held a commission as captain in a regiment of cavalry, and was endowed with many qualities which fit a man to be a soldier. I regretted that I had placed myself in his way, and I hoped by removing myself from the army, that the interest of my family would be united to further his advancement when an opportunity might offer.

I next took a view of politics. At that time the duke of Wellington had just succeeded Mr. Canning, and I had been disgusted and exasperated by what I still consider the betrayal of Portugal into the hands of Don Miguel, for continental purposes.[7] My last attachment to the Tory

---

7   Arthur Wellesley, the Duke of Wellington, became Prime Minister in 1828, but it was not an immediate succession: the Viscount Goderich served a very short 144-day term following the death of George Canning. Perceval had been stationed in Portugal in the year leading up to the Portuguese Civil War, a war of succession that followed the 1826 death of King João VI. João's eldest son, Pedro, was Emperor of the newly independent Brazil, and thus abdicated the throne to his seven-year-old daughter, now Queen Maria II of Portugal. His younger brother Miguel, an exiled absolutist rebel, was to act as regent if he would follow the nation's non-absolutist constitution. But Miguel claimed

party, and to the pride of being an Englishman, were then severed.[8] I had thought my country upright, noble, and generous, and that party honest and honourable. I now despised the one, and began to hate and fear the other. Holding his conduct to have been dishonourable in respect of Portugal, I was not surprised at the Duke's change of policy in yielding the Roman Catholic question to the Irish papists, but I was alarmed by the tone of his government, opposing the desire of the nation for reform, after that fatal blow to our Protestant institutions, and I conceived it but too possible that he might have the idea of putting down the will of the people by the bayonet; and if that struggle come, thought I, I should like to be free to choose my side, if it be agreeable to the will of God that I should interfere at all.

I was also strongly persuaded that the time of the end was at hand, and that God was about to visit the nations with his plagues, his promises having been rejected; and finding in Scripture an exhortation to his people to come out in those days from the profane, and to flee to the mountains, &c., &c., I reflected whether the words had not a practical, as well as a figurative application, and I deemed it right to place myself at liberty to act as I might be enlightened.

So, seeking liberty, I fell into confinement; seeking to serve the Almighty, I disgraced his worship and my own name. During the period that I was under personal

---

the throne and overthrew the constitution, claiming absolute power. At the conclusion of the war, in 1834, Maria would be re-throned.

8 The Tory party, which evolved into today's Conservative Party, tended to represent the upper classes and served in opposition to the more reform-minded Whigs. Under the Duke of Wellington, the Tories became more moderate. Among Wellington's policies was the passage of the Catholic Emancipation Act, to which Perceval refers below. The Act allowed Catholics to sit on Parliament.

restraint, my brother left the army, the duke of Wellington and his colleagues resigned, and were succeeded by a Whig administration; and when the cholera visited my country, I was preserved from it.[9] "It came not nigh my dwelling."[10] My own mind also had undergone a complete change in its views of the Christian faith, principle, and duty, and God knows my courage was submitted to severe trial.

---

9   The first English outbreak of cholera began in 1831. That year, it killed over 31,000 people in England, Wales, and Scotland.

10   Perceval appears to reference Psalm 91, which states that "He that dwelleth in the secret place of the Most High" will be preserved from, among other things, "the pestilence that walketh in darkness" and "the destruction that wasteth at noonday."

CHAPTER IV

Now, my readers, come with me to Oxford. I have stated
that I imagined I had found peace and triumph in the
doctrines of the evangelical preachers. I add, and it follows
of course, joy unutterable and full of glory. At first this was
the case. In Dublin, where the light of these doctrines first
broke in upon me with force sufficient to give decision to my
conduct I found in society individuals of congenial thought;
and here my own conduct was one series of devotion to
supposed religious duties and to religious enquiry. I felt
endued with a new nature, and with power to overcome
all those habits, which had most vexed me during my life.
In boldness of conduct—and of speech—in activity—in
diligence, and in purity of mind, I conceived I saw the fruits
of a new life, the evidences of the gifts of the Holy Spirit.
My mind and conduct were for the first time consistent with
each other; but when I returned to England, where I stood
alone, amongst society, and amongst officers, gentlemanly
and moderate, but indifferent to spiritual truths, and
inclined to turn *religion* or too much religion into ridicule,
I felt first puzzled, then undecided, then mistrustful of

myself, then mistrustful of my call to be a disciple of Christ Jesus,—I became lukewarm,—I became inconsistent—I fell into sin—I expected to have been kept from sin by the Holy Spirit—*that* was my idea of salvation—*that* I understood was the gift promised to me in the gospel. Now at times, I feared that I was a cast away—at times, I threw away all fear, in bold, but contrite reliance on the pledged word of the Almighty, for on that alone I fancied I had *relied*; therefore when I left the army, I desired in my own mind to retire to study at Dublin, which I called *my cradle in the Spirit*, because there I might unite society with study, and be corroborated in practice by the example of the zealous churchmen in that city. Religion is not amongst them a matter of form and ceremony, it is *the motive and end of their life*. My duty to my mother, however, and my attachment to England, determined me to choose an English university, and a hope of acquiring habits of *regularity*, made me fix on Oxford. I was pleased with my choice. The order, the quiet, the cleanliness, the beautiful simplicity of character I met with there—the majesty, the elegance, the antiquity of the buildings, the variety of their architecture, their solidity, their preservation, with all the means of study, repose, and reflection, enchanted me. I only regretted that I had not retired from a military life earlier. I only wanted, as I thought, a wife to add to my tranquillity. The evangelical doctrines I put faith in having at that time very few preachers in the church, I often frequented the Baptist and Independent meeting-houses, to hear their preachers. Soon after entering Oxford, I attended a dissenting chapel.[11] But being warned of the offence I might give to the authorities, by continuing such a course, I gave it up after my matriculation; and then went to a church where

---

11   A chapel that refused the teachings of the Church of England.

a gentleman of the name of Bulteel preached in a vehement manner doctrines then almost peculiar to himself, and in the highest degree Calvinistic.[12] On setting out for the University, I had been greatly oppressed by the fear that I should find no communion of spirit with any persons there, of my own condition. By the side of an old man's sick bed, to whose room I had been introduced by the clergyman of the parish, a friend of one of my brothers, I first met with one of the young Calvinists, who formed part of this gentleman's congregation; and he introduced me to the society of his friends, who were for the most part young men, and became my chief acquaintance. I looked upon this then as a signal instance of the Divine protection and goodness. I can now hardly forbear alluding to it with levity, as if the Almighty had said, *"if he desires it he shall have plenty."*[13] I still feel happy, in that old Bradley, (who had put on mourning at my father's death, though he knew him not,) a few days before his own death, understood that one of my father's sons had attended upon him.

About the middle of June, news came to Oxford of the extraordinary occurrences at Row and at Port Glasgow.[14]

---

12   Henry Bulteel was an Anglican preacher removed from the church due to his radical positions and his criticisms of the church. He would later be connected with the Catholic Apostolic Church, which appears in Perceval's narrative shortly.

13   Perceval may be joking about Proverbs 28:19, which says, "He that tilleth his land shall have plenty of bread: but he that followeth after vain *persons* shall have poverty enough"—i.e., plenty of nothing.

14   Row (now Rhu) and Port Glasgow are Scottish towns that lie across from one another on the river Clyde, slightly downriver from Glasgow. In 1830, Mary Campbell, a Row woman swept up in the religious fervor of a revivalist moment, was seized with the Holy Spirit and began speaking in tongues. In Port Glasgow, the apparently dying Margaret Macdonald was commanded by her prayerful brother to obey Psalm 20 and "Arise, and stand upright." She did so. The brother then wrote to Campbell, herself ill, commanding her

One evening I had crossed the river from the Christ Church meadows, and walking down the bank, through the fields on the opposite side, with two or three companions, our conversation turned on that subject: one said, if it were not for my books and other property in Oxford, I should go to Scotland to make inquiry. I replied, if I thought it true, I would sell my books and clothes if they were all that I had, to pay for my journey. The tidings were, however, so contradictory, that I did not credit the report.

It may be as well to remark here, that I had for many years often fasted, and had lately added to this discipline, watching accompanied with prayer. It was my delight to wake in the night to pray, according to the example of David—"at midnight also will I praise Thee."[15] On two occasions previous to my arrival at Oxford, during earnest prayer, I had seen visions, each of which shortly after I saw them I found were pictures of what *came to pass in reality*, though with certain variations; which I account for by my disobedience to the spirit of the vision. You do not understand this, my reader, nor do I.

I cannot now enter into a detail of these visions nor of my experiences under them. Suffice it to say, I was expecting

---

to do the same. She wrote, "when I came to the command to arise, it came home with a power which no words can describe; it was felt to be indeed the voice of Christ; it was such a voice as could not be resisted. A mighty power was instantaneously exerted upon me: I felt as if I had been lifted from off the earth, and all my diseases were taken from off me at the voice of Christ. I was verily made in a moment to stand upon my feet, leap and walk, sing and rejoice." Faith healings, speaking in tongues, and general prophesizing continued. The preacher Edward Irving was charged with heresy and thrown out of the Church of Scotland, but took the lead of a new church. Known sometimes as the Irvingites and sometimes as the Holy Catholic Apostolic Church, the organization grew, eventually incorporating a number of apostles—including Perceval's older brother Spencer.

15   Psalm 119:62.

the fulfilment of the divine prophecies, concerning the end of the world, or the coming of the Lord, and as I could see no reason but want of faith, for the absence from the church of the original gifts of the Holy Ghost, so, such experience as I had here had confirmed me in my expectation.

CHAPTER V

I LEFT OXFORD IN JULY, with the intention of proceeding to Ireland by Liverpool, on a long promised visit to one of my relations. Whilst preparing for my departure I met in London at my bankers, Mr. H. D., a gentleman who has since received the title of Evangelist, from the supposed inspired teachers of the late Mr. Irving's congregation. He gave me new information concerning the extraordinary manifestations at Row, and at Port Glasgow; and, at my desire, a letter of introduction to a young Scotch minister, who, having been thither, had returned convinced of the reality of the miracles.[16] My conversations with these two gentlemen, determined me to proceed northward to make inquiry, and to take shipping afterwards from the Clyde for Belfast.[17]

On my way, I visited my younger brother, residing at that time with his newly married wife at Sheffield. I passed a day or two with a fellow-collegian at Leeds. I passed through

---

16   See note 14.

17   The River Clyde connects Glasgow with the sea between Scotland and Ireland.

the principal manufacturing towns to Manchester, thence to Chester. I proceeded to Liverpool, and thence through the lake scenery of Westmoreland to Carlisle. Here I bid adieu to England, and arrived in Glasgow about September. In Glasgow I procured a few pamphlets then current, on the nature of the new miracles, and then descended the river, to Greenock, a town below Port Glasgow, from which place next morning I crossed over to Row, provided with a letter of introduction to Mr. Campbell the minister of Row, and also the chief preacher in those parts of the doctrines then denominated the "Row Heresy." This amiable, and I hope I may truly add godly, man received me kindly, and begged me to abide in his house, so long as I was inclined to make inquiry into the opinions of his followers.

By his means I became acquainted with Mr. Lusk, Mr. Erskine, the M'Donalds, Mary Campbell, and many others. From that which I heard, read, and saw, I soon became almost a convert. The effect then may be readily imagined which was produced on a highly excited and enthusiastic mind, by the awful thought that I was abiding in the presence and company of persons, in all probability moved and speaking by the Holy Ghost. One afternoon at Row, in the house of a gentleman, where I was at luncheon, I was first called out to see one of the inspired ladies, who had left the table and desired to speak to me, under the impression that she was commanded to address me. She was a plain slender young woman, pitted with the small pox.[18] I attended her in the drawing room, and when I was alone with her, with her arm raised and moving to a kind of serious measure, she addressed me in clear and angelic notes, with sounds like these. *"Hola mi hastos, Hola mi hastos, disca capita crustos bus-*

---

18 Smallpox left recognizable scarring on the face.

tos," &c. &c. &c. She then cried out "and he led them out to Bethany and said, Tarry ye in Jerusalem until ye are indued with power from on high."[19]

I have always felt irresistibly inclined to laugh under those circumstances which for the sake of prudence and common sense required of me the utmost outward show of gravity. So in this instance, it was with the greatest difficulty that I could command my features. At the conclusion, I asked the meaning of what I had heard. I understood that the lady thought she had been addressing me by the order of the Holy Spirit, but that she could not explain to what her words alluded. "She thought that *I* was to understand," or words to that effect. I could not help being awed; the sounds, the tone, the action, were most impressive. I felt that it was either an awful truth, or a dreadful and damnable delusion. I returned to the table where I sat down in silence. A lady on my right hand side spoke to me a few sentences which I answered, and then again I was silent, pondering in my own heart what might be the meaning of the words I had heard, if true, and how I was to obtain a decided explanation of them. Whether the command to "tarry in Jerusalem," referred to my remaining amongst the inspired persons in that neighbourhood, or to a state of peace and confidence of mind. Whilst thus reflecting, a new and wonderful sensation came upon me: from my head downwards through my whole frame, I felt a spirit or a humour[20] shedding its benign influence, the effect of which was that of the most *cheerful, mild, and grateful peace and quiet.* The words it suggested to me were, "Like to the dew of Hermon," &c. &c.[21] I do not

---

19   The latter is from Luke 24:49.

20   Bodily fluid whose fluctuations are responsible for health and mood.

21   Psalm 133:3.

remember ever having felt such, and with inward joy and pleasure I thought I recognized the marvellous work of the Almighty. I now suspect that it might have been the effect of excitement on a nervous system already undermined.[22] Yet I look back with pleasure and satisfaction on my recollection of those hours. A mind so harassed, so tortured as mine had been for many years, may well be pardoned for being deceived, by so *sensible* a delusion; by a Pandora bringing in her box a medicine so suited apparently to my complaint, and so delightful. If a doubt suggested itself, I might naturally reply in the spirit of Camoens, "*Ainda eu imagino, em ser contento?*" Am I yet only imagining when I *am* happy?[23]

After the party at that house had broken up and we were walking into Row, the lady who had addressed me, joined me, and begged that I would not take any thing that she had said to me, to bind me to remain there or in any one particular place. She was anxious lest I might be misled, and acknowledged that she did not understand the purport of the message. I then asked her if she was sure that she had faithfully discharged her mission, and had not withheld any part of the communication she had been inspired to make to me; for in her manner to me, there had appeared a want of freedom of action, as if the mind misgave itself concerning its illuminations, not daring to do or to say all it was prompted to. She was not aware that she had concealed any thing. I think it was this afternoon that we proceeded to the beach to wait for a steam packet, in which the ladies and Mr. Erskine were to pass over to Port Glasgow. No steam

---

22 Medical thought at this time held that nerves could be literally, not just figuratively, excited—as in vibrated or subject to physical strain in times of high emotion.

23 Luís de Camões (also known as Camoëns) was a sixteenth-century Portuguese poet.

packet came, owing either to foul weather, or to a change in the regulations. It was then raining, and on finding the ladies exposed to the weather, I suggested the propriety of taking shelter, but I found a pause I could not account for, until it was explained to me, that, Mr. Erskine, one of their leaders, had an impression that a steam boat would come. I was therefore obliged to leave the party, who were leaning upon this strange persuasion, to such protection as their umbrellas afforded them; I could not withstand the ridicule excited in my mind by an elderly gentleman thus misleading his flock; for I was convinced that he was mistaken in this instance at least, though I had little question of the doctrines he supported being true. I need not add that they were disappointed.

After this day, I attended the meeting of the followers of the church at Port Glasgow. Here I heard again a manifestation of tongues, and the scriptures read with an utterance preternatural, and requiring great assurance to practise, because so extraordinary. I never attended these meetings without great conflict of mind, and afterwards depression. I had an anxiety working in me, and a bond pressing down heavy on me. I knew not what I was to do; my mind was in the dark, yet I wanted to be taking *an active* part. The sounds I heard were at times beautiful in the extreme, resembling the Greek language; at times they were awfully sublime and grand, and gave me a full perception of that idea; "the Word was with God, and the Word was God:"[24] at times the tone of them querulous and almost ridiculous.

One evening, after having attended one of these meetings, I retired to the inn at Port Glasgow, and feeling not disposed to go so early to bed, I went into the travellers'

---

24   John 1:1.

room, and ordered a glass of whiskey. I was soon after joined by a Scotch gentleman, who also ordered some whiskey, with which, from his appearance, he was far better acquainted than myself. This kind of frolicsome squire or laird I shrank from, having a most hearty dislike to riot and extravagance. The more, however, my nature shrank from him, the more need I imagined he had of Christian charity and instruction. We fell into conversation, and I was very much afflicted, when we descanted on religious subjects, and on the reported miracles in the neighbourhood, at the broken-hearted manner in which my companion confessed and complained of his own weakness, and declared for himself he was unable to be a Christian—as for himself, he was sure that he had no kindred with Christ. During my conversation, I was dwelling intently upon the means most likely to quicken him to a sense of shame and hope; and looking, though despondingly, to be guided by the Holy Spirit in my argument. I suffered a deep internal struggle—I seemed guided to I knew not what: at last, I flung myself back, as it were, in the arms of the Lord; and opening my mouth, I sang without premeditation, in beautiful tones, that affected my mind greatly, and in measure like to an anthem, "kindred with Christ! bone of his bone, and flesh of his flesh!"[25] The manner was that of expostulation for want of faith, of encouragement and consolation. I sang a few more sentences in the same apparently inspired manner, but without premeditation; I forget them, but I recollect after a short but animated conversation, the gentleman, greatly touched and awed into compunction, rose up and kissed me, declaring that he trusted there were still hopes for him; and he left me, promising to attend one of the meetings next day.

---

25   Ephesians 5:30.

I could mention several instances of the same kind, when the power of the Spirit came upon me, and, opening my mouth, sang in beautiful tones words of purity, kindness, and consolation. I was subdued and humbled; it was not my doing—the words, the ideas even, were wholly unthought of by me, or at least I was unconscious of thinking of them

Et, quoniam Deus ora movet, sequar ora moventem

Rite Deum———[26]

Ovid's description of the inspiration of Pythagoras tallied with my experience. This voice was given me, but I was not the master of it; I was but the instrument. I could not use it at my own command, but solely at the command of the Spirit that guided me. On another occasion, I was going to call for the first time on Mary Campbell, had crossed the ferry over the lake, and was proceeding along the shore on the opposite side, when I passed a party of ladies with one gentleman. I felt impelled in the Spirit to give a message to them. I shrank from doing so, conceiving it to be a delusion, but again fearing that I was grieving the Spirit, and proving ungrateful through my timidity before man, I summoned resolution, and addressed a few words of scripture to the lady and gentleman in front of the party when they came up. The lady, with great delicacy and command, questioned me as to what I meant, without showing offence or confusion. I replied that I did not know to what the words alluded, but that I believed I had been desired to utter them. I never could tell why. I afterwards conversed with the lady, who was acquainted with my eldest brother's wife's family. I learned that the gentleman walking with her was apparently

---

26 In Ovid's *Metamorphoses* Book XV, he writes as Pythagoras: "Now, since a god moves my lips, I will follow, with due rite, the god who moves those lips." (Translated by A.S. Kline.)

reforming, from having been of an unthinking and wild character; and, soon after, I was told that one of the young ladies behind recognised me, having sailed across the Clyde in the same steam-boat with myself; on that day we had conversed together on the subject of the manifestations at Port Glasgow and Row. I had argued with her on the possibility and apparent probability of them, and she had expressed her desire to know the result of my inquiries. I was then able to tell her, that I not only believed in the reality of the miracles, but that I imagined I had myself been a subject of them.

At morning service in Mr. Campbell's church, one Sunday, I was led to open my mouth, and sing a part of a psalm, at a time when the rest of the congregation were at peace, and whilst Mr. Campbell was preparing to preach. *I mistrusted the guidance, I knew not what then to do*; but after inward conflict, whilst Mr. Campbell was actually preaching, I gained confidence to chant two verses of *another psalm*. I was immediately below, and behind, the pulpit. Mr. Campbell descended from it to dissuade me, and begged me not to continue. I told him quietly, "I had done." The power had left me. I knew not whether I had done right or wrong; I only knew the power was not mine, and from its nature, as evidenced to my own feelings, I concluded it divine: afterwards, in a conversation with Mary Campbell, I understood that which is written by St. Paul, that we are not to speak all together, but to command the spirits; for that God is not a God of confusion, but of order.

Afterwards I assisted Mr. Campbell to write out his apology, and attended him to Dumbarton,[27] where he was condemned by a set of crabbed old Presbyterians calling themselves a synod, presided over by a person called

27 Another Scottish town on the banks of the Clyde.

"Moderator," a stout, mild, rosy-faced man, the only gentleman amongst them.[28] Whilst waiting for their arrival,
and for the opening of the church doors, I walked amongst
the graves with Macdonald, one of two brothers who had
originated these doctrines, and whose sister had been raised
miraculously from a bed of sickness.[29] He told me that since
he had been converted, he had *lived as in a new life*—moved
by a life that dwelt in him. The same young man, or his
brother, whilst the mock trial was going on, rushed out
of the church, crying out words with a loud voice to this
effect, "Come out of her, come out of her, my people."[30] I do
not recollect the exact speech; he was red in the face. My
impression at the time was that he was misled, not in faith,
but in so giving utterance to it.

---

28   The Church of Scotland is a Presbyterian church, and a synod is a church
court. The group was likely convened to reach a judgment on the Irvingite
movement.

29   This is Margaret, introduced in note 14.

30   Revelations 18:4. The "her" is Babylon: "Babylon the great is fallen, is
fallen, and is become the habitation of devils, and the hold of every foul spirit,
and a cage of every unclean and hateful bird. For all nations have drunk of
the wine of the wrath of her fornication, and the kings of the earth have
committed fornication with her, and the merchants of the earth are waxed
rich through the abundance of her delicacies. And I heard another voice from
heaven, saying, Come out of her, my people, that ye be not partakers of her
sins, and that ye receive not of her plagues. For her sins have reached unto
heaven, and God hath remembered her iniquities."

CHAPTER VI

I WILL NOT NOW DWELL any more upon these particulars: suffice it to say, I left the manse at Row, *in my own imagination*, a living instance of the Holy Ghost operating in man,—full of courage, confidence, peace, and rapture, like a glowing flame, but still and submissive. Such, I say, was the state of my feeling in the life of that Spirit; but in the flesh I was anxious, lest I should be betrayed into error by a false zeal, or by false directions, so as to turn that power to ridicule, by attempting miracles, uncommanded, or by conduct out of order; at the same time, I was alarmed, lest, mistaking a fear of man for a love of order, I might quench the Holy Spirit working within me. I knew it was in my power to refuse to obey the Spirit's guidance, but not to *command* its utterance. At the same time, I knew the power of utterance was often upon me, when I considered it out of season and place to make use of it. This disturbed me, because others had told me, they could not resist the power, when it came upon them! Mr. Campbell, at my departure seemed to fear for me, that I might be misled, and expressed his anxiety; I was conscious of danger and difficulty, but I hoped what had been begun without me, would be perfected in me, despite even of myself.

I recollect one night at Mr. Campbell's, whilst reading the Scriptures, I was directed to read, or to expound to him, certain passages, which I declined doing, as out of place and presumptuous. He went out of the room, and the Spirit then guided me to several chapters and verses, containing *warnings*, reproof, and menaces; particularly to the first chapter of Jeremiah, verse 17. "Be not dismayed at their faces, lest I confound thee before them;" *where the Prophet is threatened with confusion if he is disobedient.* These threats were applied to me, I was alarmed, and when Mr. Campbell re-entered, I acknowledged the inward working of the Spirit, and stated to him my opinions concerning the "*identity of the church with the Lord,*" which I had been afraid to mention before, lest I might be charged with enthusiasm. At Dublin again, after a conflict of a similar nature, when I had left a gentleman's house to go I knew not whither, I was made to open the Old Testament, and in the books of the law, the twenty-eighth chapter of Deuteronomy was pointed out to me to read, containing the curses, that I should be cursed in my family, in going out and coming in, &c., "and the Lord shall smite thee with madness and blindness and astonishment of heart." The passages were applied to me, and I was shocked, and yet I could not see *how it could be true*, seeing *the Lord had promised to keep me*, as well as to save me and convert me.

Before I quitted Row, however, I had suspected that a new power had been conferred on me, of discerning the spirits that spoke in men around me, by their tone, and the effect of the utterance upon my nervous organs. This was a new field of observation to me when I left Scotland, and I considered it might be, if not a delusion, a beneficial guard against any spiritual enemy; but when I came to Ireland, in addition to the power of discerning evil in others, I fancied that I had the power to discern evil in myself, and to know by the sensation on my palate, throat, and hearing, whether I was speaking in accordance with the will of God, or against his will, and consequently against the laws of nature. I now attribute this sensation in a great measure to extreme nervous excitement, but at that time it led to the destruction of my new formed peace, and ultimately to my ruin. For I was conscious that I spoke often with bodily pain, in reply to trivial or religious questions, and at the same time I could not *but answer* or hold my tongue. If I held my tongue, I was embarrassed, and I caused pain and displeasure and suspicion to others, which I could not believe consistent with Christian charity. Yet I must either hold my tongue, or speak as I was guided, or speak my own thoughts; and when no guidance came, I would, at times, stumble upon broken sentences, stammer, and prove ridiculous, opening my mouth to obey a guidance which failed me before I finished a sentence, at times even before I commenced. Still less could I think it my duty to make my mission ridiculous: yet in speaking my own thoughts as I then termed them, I groaned in spirit and grieved, suffering actually bodily pain, and fearing that I was guilty of, and accusing myself of, the grossest ingratitude in rebelling even against the law of nature, and not only against the Holy Spirit, to whom I was indebted for such great mercies, and miraculous graces. This trouble of mind increased upon me towards the end of November, and the commencement of December, and was the most active inward cause of all my misfortunes.

I landed at Belfast, where I halted for the Sunday, and then proceeded to Dublin, bearing witness on my way to what I had witnessed in Scotland: on the road I recollect I lost a Hebrew Bible,—I met, as I had expected and desired, in Dublin, a gentleman who had offered me a curacy in Somersetshire.[31] To him I related my convictions, prepared to meet with a withdrawal of his offer in consequence, which however did not follow. My kind friend appeared willing to look upon my enthusiasm with indulgence, and to leave it with the bishop, whom he invited me to meet near Bristol, to decide if it was too strong to allow of ordination into the church. I was, however, otherwise guided, and, after passing a few days in Dublin, I proceeded to fulfil an engagement in Queen's County, and from thence journeyed beyond Limerick to visit a schoolfellow, a zealous clergyman acting as curate in a small Irish town.[32] On my way there, I spent a night or two at the house of a protestant clergyman near *Roscrea*, to whom I had a letter of introduction; he was an enthusiast of the evangelical school; he begged me to accompany him next day to a meeting at Nenagh, at which he begged me to assist.[33] I assented with some difficulty, because I had not yet had any distinct calling or command to appear publicly. Although I often desired to have a way opened for me, yet I feared to be trespassing on paths not prepared for me by the Lord; for all the guidance I had hitherto received, after my conversation with Mary Campbell, *tended to the strictest order* and obedience to the ordinances of the church. I did however accept the invitation to speak conditionally; an express condition was, that I should confine myself to general subjects, and not be supposed to give an unqualified support to a society not acting in strict union

31 A position working for the church in the south-west of England.

32 Perceval was traveling from Dublin toward the western coast of Ireland.

33 Small towns in the west of Ireland.

with and subordination to the established church. I went to the meeting completely unprepared. I decided when there, what line of argument to adopt, in conformity with the will of my *singular inspiration*, and being at a loss to know how to support my argument with texts, and doubting the will or mistrusting the power of the Spirit, to speak through me uninterruptedly, I applied inwardly for guidance; and the Spirit, moving my arms and fingers, opened for me my Bible in distinct places, one after the other, supplying me in each place with a passage in regular connexion with my line of argument. According to these I spoke.

I mention these facts, to show the reasonableness, if I may so call it, of my lunacy, *if it was entirely lunacy*; to speak more clearly, to show the reality of the *existence of that power*, by the abuse or use of which, I became insane. If by the abuse of it, because the Lord confounded me for my disobedience; if by the use of it, because, though real, it was a spirit of delusion.

After paying another visit, near Limerick, I returned to Dublin about the third week in November. I there met with two individuals who had been at Row, and I was tempted to protract my stay until they returned to Scotland. My mind was no longer quiet. Incapable of speaking even on trivial subjects, without internal rebuke and misgiving, accompanied with real nervous pain, uncertain what was the origin of this, or the end pointed to, I felt inclined often to give up all care in religion, exhausted, weary, and broken hearted. One Friday evening whilst returning from a family dinner, after which I had been arguing with a friend, under my usual sense of perplexity and inward struggle, as I passed round by the college towards the bridge, I was assailed by a woman of the town, as is their custom, to whom I spoke, with a heavy heart, in the language of Scripture warning her of her danger. She left me, and five minutes after that, another coming alongside of me, led me away to my destruction. My confinement, my sense of shame, of ingratitude, of remorse, my continual accusation of myself, that I did not feel the extent of my crime, of my guilt in bringing disrepute on doctrines I was persuaded came from the Holy Spirit, the abiding presence of this guiding power influencing my actions, and awing my mind, added to the subtle effects of mercury upon the humours of my body, during the use of which I had the imprudence to expose my frame to draughts, whilst washing for a long time, every morning, my whole person in cold water, at that inclement season of the year; these causes all combined, could hardly fail to effect the ruin of my mind; but they were joined with others which I will mention in order in the next chapter.[34]

My reader, I have had great difficulty to get even thus far, but, if after this you meet with more irregularity and abruptness of style, and change of manner, recollect how painful a task I am engaged in, and pass it over.

---

34 Perceval would have taken mercury to treat a case of syphilis that he believed he received from the sex worker. His attribution of his insanity to both psychological and physical causes is very typical of nineteenth-century accounts.

CHAPTER VII

I WAS INTIMATELY ACQUAINTED with the family of an officer residing in Dublin, of moderate and religious principles. He had constantly called on me during my illness, and when I became convalescent he invited me to pass the Sunday with him, having observed how my imagination was preying upon my mind, and fearing for me, for I had related to him the strange guidances and sensations to which I was become familiar, hoping that a cheerful evening with my old friends might be of advantage to me; and I accepted the invitation. It was about the 19th of December. Unfortunately I would have it that I was to speak in an unknown tongue, and to do other marvellous feats before this family, in order to convince them of the truth of the Row doctrines, preparatory to my departure for England, which I was wild enough to fix for the end of the week. For I conceived that my speedy restoration from the illness which had recently afflicted me, was the effect of a miraculous blessing on the means made use of, and a great mercy; and now I was well, I imagined it was a trial of my faith, and so it was, whether I should still submit to the regimen and prescriptions of my physician, or, by kicking the stool on which I had been standing from under my feet, show the power that had healed me, and at the same time my faith in that power. I say this was indeed a trial of my faith, in two senses, for it was a trial of the strength of my delusion, and of my reasonable understanding: of my real faith, which I then called human fear; and of my false faith, which I then called trust in God. It is contemptible and ridiculous, but when night came and I had to decide, I split the difference by taking half the dose that my physician had ordered me. The truth is, that I doubted my delusions, and I doubted my physician. Had my mind been clear, I might have been acting wisely, and with peace of mind; but my mind being confused, this trifling incident added to my confusion, and, my conscience being doubtful, to my imagined guilt. All this contributed to my disturbance that wretched night.

I say that I imagined I was to speak in an unknown tongue, and perform other signs before my worthy friend's household. And this, though a delusion, is but a delusion of this world, where the worthless are putting themselves forward continually as God's truest servants: the most ignorant are the most presumptuous. This delusion, however, counterbalanced all the beneficial effects of their society, for I was in a state of great excitement, both at my own feelings, that urged and led me to attempt utterances and singing, &c. &c., and at their alarm and opposition. It is said in Scripture that the disciples should *do wonders*, and amongst other wonders, more harmless, it came into my head, I am told, to put my hand *into the fire*, persuaded that I might draw it out unhurt. I was either dissuaded or prevented from doing this. During the evening I discovered I had not brought my pocket-handkerchief. My friend

Captain —— sent for one of his, it was of red silk; the impression came on my mind that it was a token of ill to me, and I exclaimed ————what have you given me? you have given me blood.[35] Conversation was going on and my words were hushed over, but I foreboded a calamity which though inevitable I could not distinctly foresee.

On retiring to sleep, I promised my host not to cry out in prayer or in hymn; that I might not disturb any of the old pensioners in the Kilmainham hospital, in a room of which my bed was prepared.[36]

In the night I awoke under the most dreadful impressions; I heard a voice addressing me, and I was made to imagine that my disobedience to the faith, in taking the medicine overnight, had not only offended the Lord, but had rendered the work of my salvation extremely difficult, by its effect upon my spirits and humours. I heard that I could only be saved now by being changed into a spiritual body; and that a great fight would take place in my mortal body between Satan and Jesus; the result of which would either be my perfection in a spiritual body, or my awaking in hell. I am not sure whether before or after this, I was now commanded to cry out aloud, for consenting to which I was immediately rebuked, as unmindful of the promise I had made to my friend. A spirit came upon me and prepared to guide me in my actions. I was lying on my back, and the spirit seemed to light on my pillow by my right ear, and to command my body. I was placed in a fatiguing attitude, resting on my feet, my knees drawn up and on my head, and made to swing my body from side to side without ceasing. In the meantime, I

35 Nineteenth-century texts often used dashes in places of names for the sake of anonymity.

36 The hospital was originally a home for retired soldiers.

heard voices without and within me, and sounds as of the clanking of iron, and the breathing of great forge bellows, and the force of flames. I understood that I was only saved by the mercy of Jesus, from seeing, as well as hearing, hell around me; and that if I were not obedient to His spirit, I should inevitably awake in hell before the morning. After some time I had a little rest, and then, actuated by the same spirit, I took a like position on the floor, where I remained, until I understood that the work of the Lord was perfected, and that now my salvation was secured; at the same time the guidance of the spirit left me, and I became in doubt what next I was to do. I understood that this provoked the Lord, as if I was affecting ignorance when I knew what I was to do, and, after some hesitation, I heard the command, to *"take your position on the floor again then,"* but I had no guidance or no perfect guidance to do so, and could not resume it. I was told, however, that my salvation depended upon my maintaining that position as well as I could until the morning; and oh! great was my joy when I perceived the first brightness of the dawn, which I could scarcely believe had arrived so early. I then retired to bed. I had imagined during the night that the fire of hell was consuming my mortal body—that the Spirit of Jesus came down to me to endure the pain thereof for me, that he might perfect in me a spiritual body to His honour and glory. I imagined that the end of this work was, that I was already in the state of one raised from the dead; and that any sin or disobedience in this body was doubly horrible and loathsome, inasmuch as it was in a body actually regenerated and clothed upon with the Holy Ghost. I imagined also that the Holy Ghost had in a special manner descended, and worked with Jesus to save me. I considered it a proof of the truth of my imaginations, when on rising, being perplexed by two different guidings that came upon me, I looked down upon my limbs which were white and of a natural colour; and again I looked down on my limbs, when one half of my frame appeared in a state of scarlet inflammation. When I went to dress, this had again subsided.

Before I rose from my bed, I understood that I was now to proceed through the world *as an angel*, under the immediate guidance of the Lord, to proclaim the tidings of his second coming. With that came an *uncertain* impression that I was to do this in an extraordinary way, and by singing—and this idea haunted me throughout my changes of insanity. I had also an uncertain impression of a like nature, that I was to go and show myself before the lord lieutenant or the General of the Forces, that I was to breakfast there, and to meet, either at the lord lieutenant's, a prince of the blood royal; or at the General's, a duke, to whom I was to proclaim the near coming of the Lord.

My guidance not being sure, and my folly or my faith not being firm enough, I reflected on Mary Campbell's advice, and determined to be guided by what appeared the natural path of duty. And, at the risk of offending the Holy Spirit and the Lord, to prefer showing my gratitude to Captain H. who had shown me so many kind attentions, and to attend his humble table. I now conceived again that I was to speak to them in an unknown tongue, and to make confessions, and to show signs and wonders: my words and ideas were to be supplied to me. I did not, however, dare to attempt any thing, for I felt no guidance, and I shrank from the ridicule of beginning to speak, and having nothing to say. My whole conduct became confused, my language ambiguous and doubtful. After breakfast, I prayed to be left alone, which was accorded with some difficulty. When alone in the breakfast room, I expected to be guided to prayer; but a spirit guided me and placed me on a chair, in a constrained position, with my head turned to *look at the clock*, the hand of which I saw proceeding to the first quarter; I understood I was to leave the position when it came to the quarter; when, however, it came to the quarter, I was anxious to be on the safe side, and I waited till it was at least half a minute past. Having done this, I was not a whit the wiser; but on the contrary, I felt that I had again offended by my want of exact punctuality, proving my want of confidence. I was then directed to lie on the floor, with my face to the ground, in an attitude of supplication and humiliation. I heard a spirit pray in me, and reason in me, and with me, and ultimately, another spirit, desiring certain gifts of the Holy Spirit to be given me, amongst which prophecy, tongues, miracles, and discernment of spirits; soon after, I was overwhelmed with a sudden and mighty conviction of my utter worthlessness; and being asked how I could expect the Lord to take me, and on what conditions I craved his favour; another spirit cried out in me, and for me, *"Lord! take me as I am."*

CHAPTER VIII

AT THAT MOMENT Captain H. entered, and I arose. His family came into the room, and I again began to be troubled with the idea that I was to make confessions to them, and to speak in an unknown tongue. I had not understanding to do either, and my conduct became very unintelligible. Capt. H. sat down to write a letter, and I attempted to make a sketch partly from memory, and partly by the guidance of the power that moved my hands, of my mother's residence. Captain H. after finishing his letter, sent for a hackney coach in which I proceeded with him to Dublin. On my way, I was tormented by the commands of what I imagined was the Holy Spirit, to say other things, which as óften as I attempted, I was fearfully rebuked for beginning in my own voice, and not in a voice given to me. These contradictory commands were the cause, now, as before, of the incoherency of my behaviour, and these imaginations formed the chief causes of my ultimate total derangement. For I was commanded to speak, on pain of dreadful torments, of provoking the wrath of the Holy Spirit, and of incurring the guilt of the grossest ingratitude; and at the same moment, whenever I attempted to speak, I was harshly and contumeliously rebuked for not using the utterance of a spirit sent to me; and when again I attempted, I still went wrong, and when I pleaded internally that I knew not what I was to do, I was accused of false-hood and deceit; and of being really unwilling to do what I was commanded. I then lost patience, and proceeded to say what I was desired pell-mell, determined to show that it was not fear or want of will that prevented me. But when I did this, I felt as formerly the pain in the nerves of my palate and throat on speaking, which convinced me that I was not only rebelling against God, but against nature; and I relapsed into an agonizing sense of hopelessness and of ingratitude.

We arrived at my hotel, when Captain ——— left me to bring in my physician, Dr. P.[37] I threw myself at the feet of my bed, endeavouring to pray. I think my physician came and again I was left alone, when, after much meditation, I prepared to go out to order a hat, and to arrange for my return to England in one of the Howth packets.[38] But, when I opened the door, I found a stout man servant on the land-ing, who told me that he was placed there to forbid my going out, by the orders of Dr. P. and my friend; on my remon-strating, he followed me into my room and stood before the door. I insisted on going out; he, on preventing me. I warned him of the danger he incurred in opposing the will of the Holy Spirit, I prayed him to let me pass, or otherwise an evil would befal him, for that I was a prophet of the Lord. He was not a whit shaken by my address, so, after again and

---

37   Dr. P would be revealed in Perceval's second narrative as Dr. Piel.

38   Howth is a village located to the east of Dublin on a peninsula reaching toward England. A packet ship sailed on a routine schedule, carrying mail and passengers.

again adjuring him, by the desire of the Spirit whose word I heard, I seized one of his arms, desiring it to wither: my words were idle, no effect followed, and I was ashamed and astonished.

Then, thought I, I have been made a fool of! But I did not on that account mistrust the doctrines by which I had been exposed to this error. The doctrines, thought I, are true; but I am mocked at by the Almighty for my disobedience to them, and at the same time, I have the guilt and the grief, of bringing discredit upon the truth, by my obedience to a spirit of mockery, or, by my disobedience to the Holy Spirit; for there were not wanting voices to suggest to me, that the reason why the miracle had failed, was, that I had not waited for the Spirit to guide my action when the word was spoken, and that I had seized the man's arm with the wrong hand. I was silent and astonished. Bed time came. I requested the man to leave me for half an hour for prayer; he did so. Before that, I think Captain H. had been to me, and had explained the reason of his being there. I went to bed, but not to sleep.

In the same manner as I have already related, voices came to desire me to say and attempt many things, which, at one time, I was to utter in the spirit of holiness; at another, in my own spirit, at another time, in another spirit; which, as surely as they were enjoined, I as surely appeared to misplace, and as surely received the most cutting and insulting reproaches for failing in. At one time, I was to sing, at another, to pray; at another, to address my attendant; at another, to ask him to come to my bed, which my sense of decorum refused; at another, to desire him to make a bed for himself on the sofa, which I counselled him to do, and which I think he declined; at last, in one of these mental conflicts, hunted in every direction, my patience gave way, and I mentally cursed the Holy Trinity. A cutting sense of my ingratitude, and deep grief, followed, with mute despair.

The voices informed me, that my conduct was owing to a spirit of mockery and blasphemy having possession of me. That as I was already the object of the special grace of the Holy Spirit, which had undertaken my salvation, by rendering me a spiritual body, after I had forfeited my hope in Jesus Christ, there was no longer hope for me in the ordinary means of faith and prayer; but, that I must, in the power of the Holy Spirit, *redeem myself* and rid myself of the spirits of blasphemy and mockery that had taken possession of me.

The way in which I was tempted to do this was by throwing myself on the top of my head backwards, and so resting on the top of my head and on my feet alone, to turn from one side to the other until I had broken my neck. I suppose by this time I was already in a state of feverish delirium, but my good sense and prudence still refused to undertake this strange action. I was then accused of faithlessness and cowardice, of fearing man more than God.

And so it was, that the means taken for my care, by my friend and the doctor, became my destruction, owing to the peculiar weaknesses of my understanding.[39] I was made to doubt my own sincerity, and to desire to prove it in spite of the presence of the domestic. Had he not been there, I might by that time have been sound asleep.

I attempted the command, the servant prevented me. I lay down contented to have proved myself willing to obey in

39 Perceval is stressing that attempts to help him—in this case, to assign someone to watch over him—were misguided. He makes similar criticisms throughout, offering first-hand experience on the best methods for caring for the insane.

spite of his presence, but now I was accused of not daring to wrestle with him unto blows. I again attempted what I was enjoined. The man seized me, I tore myself from him, telling him it was necessary for my salvation; he left me and went down stairs. I then tried to perform what I had begun; but now I found, either that I could not so jerk myself round on my head, or that my fear of breaking my neck was really too strong for my faith. In that case I then certainly mocked, for my efforts were not sincere.

When I undertook this action, I imagined that if I performed it in the power of the Holy Spirit, no harm would result to me, but that if I threw myself round to the right in my own strength, I might break my neck and die, but that I should be raised again immediately to fulfil my mission. I had therefore no design to destroy myself; but, I have often conjectured since, that God in his mercy may have meditated my self-destruction to save me from the horrors he foresaw preparing for me: they were great and intolerable, shocking in themselves, more shocking in my abandonment; I awoke from them as from the grave, to be cut off from all my tenderest ties.[40]

Failing in my attempts, I was directed to expectorate[41] violently, in order to get rid of my two formidable enemies; and then again I was told to drink water, and that the Almighty was satisfied; but that if I was not satisfied (neither could I be sincerely, for I knew I had not fulfilled his commands), I was to take my position again; I did so; my attendant came up with an assistant and they forced me into

---

40 Perceval is foreshadowing the conclusion of his asylum care, when he found himself estranged from the family he felt had betrayed him.

41 Spit.

AGENTS WANTED

*To Canvass for this work. Specimen sheets furnished and
full information given on application.*

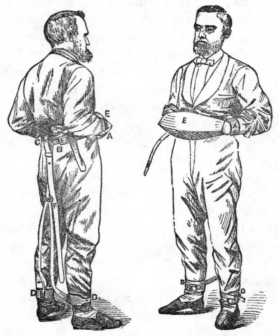

Sells Rapidly.   Liberal inducements offered.

Address   MOSES SWAN,
Hoosick Falls, N. Y.

A schematic of a straitjacket
from an 1874 asylum exposé by Moses Swan.

a straight waistcoat.[42] Even then I again tried to resume the position to which I was again challenged. They then tied my legs to the bed-posts, and so secured me.

Let me remark, how I became the victim of so absurd a delusion, yet having so much sense and reflection left to me. The spirits which at first spoke in my hearing, or addressed me at Row and Port Glasgow, and afterwards spoke in me and moved me; which subsequently in Ireland I heard talking to me, and communing with me invisible; had an utterance so pure, so touching, so beautiful, that I could not but believe them divine. They spake also in accordance with the word of life; they directed me in paths of peace, obedience, and humility; they flattered me even in my desire to adhere to the church establishment, and not to break the visible unity of the church; they came upon me to teach me method and order; they guided my hand to write in letters unusual to me; in so many ways they were attested, as spirits of good and of wisdom, that, now even, I dare not deny the possibility of disobedience to them, not my obedience, having caused me to be confounded, which was forewarned me in Scotland. But when I had thrown myself away, *and I was thrown away*, I was decoyed and separated from Jesus, the rock of a Christian's salvation, by my reliance on these sounds. For, as it is written, the word of the Lord came to the prophets, to Isaiah, &c. &c. when the voice came to *me*, I received that voice as the word of the Lord; and the rather, because, when I first heard it, it was like that Elijah describes, "a still small voice," and the directions of that voice were like the rest of my experiences at first, which were to my apparent

---

42   A straitjacket. Such mechanisms for restraint were already criticized at the time, but they were often used in the case of patients deemed violent or suicidal.

good, and for my instruction.[43] Now, afterwards that voice weaned me from my reliance upon the blood of Jesus—even through my hope in the mercies of Jesus, telling me that I could no longer be saved by the ordained means of faith, hope, and charity; but by the special interference of the Holy Ghost, and fellow-working of Jesus in me, to transform my body; this I admitted, though I could not understand it, on the authority of the spirits communing with me, the rather because it showed forth the mercies of Jesus the more extraordinarily. Thus having been once decoyed from looking up to the cross of Jesus as my only hope of salvation, it became comparatively easy for the same power, by the same means, to suggest to me a new necessity for an unusual act on my part to save me, when I had forfeited my new state of grace. For at that time I was, in all probability, already in a state of feverish delirium.

However, I did not give yet entire credit to these voices, or at least, I still exercised in certain respects my judgment and suspicion upon them, recollecting the example and warning of Mary Campbell. Particularly, finding the tones vary, I asked which is the voice of God? but my suspicions were soon lulled again, and my objections in part put down, by the suggestion that I heard the voices of the three members of the Holy Trinity, and afterwards those of the spirits of God sent to me to command me in His name.

I perished from an habitual error of mind, common to many believers, and particularly to our brethren the Roman Catholics. That *of fearing to doubt, and of taking the guilt of doubt* upon my conscience; the consequence of this is, want of candour and of real sincerity; because we force ourselves to say we believe what we do not believe, because we think

---

43   Isaiah and Elijah were Israelite prophets.

doubt sinful. Whereas we cannot control our doubts, which can only be corrected by information. To reject persuasion wilfully is one crime; but to declare wilfully that we believe what we doubt, or presumptuously that our doubts are wilful, is another.

CHAPTER IX

THE NEXT DAY, or the day after, Dr. P. entered my room with another doctor. When they came to my bed-side, I was silent. I was unable to explain myself to them, because I knew that Dr. P. was reputed to be an Unitarian, and therefore I conceived it impossible to make him credit the supernatural voices and agency under which I acted.[44] His companion seemed so stupid, and so like a man of the world of a common and vague stamp of mind, that I thought it perhaps still more hopeless to address him.

They remained about five or ten minutes on the left-hand side of my bed, and then went away. I have since learned, that this wise second to Dr. P. was a lunatic doctor, celebrated in Dublin. And to that, in part, I cannot help attributing my subsequent misfortunes.[45] I imagine that had Dr. P. acted on his own sound judgment, he would never

---

44   As a Unitarian, Dr. Piel rejected the idea of the Holy Trinity, to which Perceval attributed the multiple voices that he was hearing.

45   The critiques that Perceval levies against "lunatic doctors" are characteristic of those throughout his life, and of many who believed that specialization divorced medical men from common sense. Lunatic doctors were particularly suspicious because they had a financial interest in depriving others of their liberty.

have allowed me, however extraordinary my complaint
might appear, to be subjected to the equally extraordinary
treatment of confinement to my bed, in nearly one position
for several days together, tied hand and foot in a straight
waistcoat, and in a small and close room. He would have
said, whatever harm may be in him, or may arrive to him
from his complaint, it cannot be greater than what will
certainly happen, if he be confined so. But having submitted
me to the treatment of a lunatic doctor, he submitted his
own judgment along with it; through that infatuation by
which so many are duped to allow these men to deal with
patients contrary to nature, law, and reason, purely because
they profess to undertake practically the care of men devoid
of reason; affecting, at the same time, that the complaint
itself is wholly wrapped up in unfathomable mystery. I
imagine, had I been treated according to nature, if under this
treatment I was restored, through much danger, to a state fit
for hazarding a journey, about the middle of January, I might
then have been recovered in less time, with less suffering,
and more perfectly from the state of derangement which
my excitement of mind, acting on a disordered system, had
brought on only for a time. But fate ordered otherwise. I was
confined in the manner above detailed; the reason of this
was the fear of violence to myself. My need of wholesome
exercise and occupation was denied. My idleness of mind
and body left me at the mercy of my delusions; my confined
position increased or caused a state of fever, which brought
on delirium; and they kept drenching my body to take away
the evil which their system was continually exciting;[46] and

---

46 Hydrotherapy was a popular "treatment" for madness, believed to cool
the overheated brain and thus soothe the mind. Just as importantly, it subjected the patient to the doctor's control.

which ultimately triumphed completely over me. My want of exercise produced a deadly torpor in the moral functions of my mind, combined with the ruin of my spirits by their diet and medicines. I foresaw a dreadful doom which I could not define, and from which, like one in a dream, I attempted in vain to run away. Inwardly I adjured my Maker, and expostulated with the voices communing with me, in me, or without me, to allow me exercise, as the only means of saving me. I addressed no one, or scarcely addressed any outwardly, partly because I considered it hopeless, without pledging myself to attempt what my obedience to divine inspiration bade me attempt—hopeless to persuade them of my divine inspiration, partly because if ever I attempted to speak, I was checked and rated by the spirits, for using my own filthy utterance, or abusing the divine utterance. Since boyhood, I had never been confined to my bed for more than two or three days, nor to my room, for so much as a week together; and on an average had never had less daily, than three hours' active exercise. Now, after a fortnight's confinement to my room, I was fastened on my bed, with the liberty of my arms and legs denied to me.

I do not know how long this continued, but I recollect when my eldest brother came to my bed side, he found me so, and many days after his arrival in Dublin I continued to be so. It is true my legs were occasionally loosed, but they were as quickly tied down again on my resuming my insane attempts, or trying to get out of bed. This I used to do for two reasons; one to get water, for which I longed, and in which I think I succeeded once, either by my own efforts, or by the servant guessing at my desire, one day after my brother's arrival; otherwise, I am afraid it is too true, I had no water to drink ever offered to me, but broth, and the most filthy medicine, that tasted like steel filings in a strong acid. Neither do I recollect receiving any solid food. I usually resisted both the administering of the broth and of the medicine, being commanded to do so, with circumstances of much spiritual insult, horror, and indelicacy, which I cannot now repeat. The other reason for which I attempted to rise out of bed, was to get to the window to see if it were true, as my tormentors told me, that all my family were there waiting to receive me, and to hail me as an obedient servant of the Lord Jesus, and a willing martyr to his glory. For when I began to lose all command of my imagination, I was made to believe, that in consequence of my disobedience and blasphemies against Jesus Christ and the Holy Spirit, the Roman Catholics in Ireland, to whom I had been ordained as an angel, being miraculously informed like the shepherds, by an angel shining in the glory of the Lord, had risen up and come to Dublin, demanding my crucifixion or my burning; that in the mean time the Almighty, provoked by my great perfidy and ingratitude, had cut short the days and revoked his counsels; had determined to visit my nation with severe plagues, and me, with all the torments he had reserved for Satan, whom even he had pardoned, glad to find one, and one only, who deserved all his everlasting plagues, and to be able thereby to pardon his immense creation.

I was the one only being to be eternally damned, alone, in multiplied bodies, and in infinite solitude and darkness and torments. I was told also that the Almighty in His three persons had descended upon earth, had entered London, and had revealed all these things to the king, who was also preparing on earth the most cruel torments for me; that my father and a sister who is now no more, had been raised from the dead, and had interceded for me, and that my relations and friends had assembled round me in Dublin, and had defended me from the violence of the mob at the sacrifice of their own lives. My friend Captain H.'s coat which occasionally lay upon my sofa, for he was constantly attending upon me, was to my delirious imagination, a proof of his murder in my defence. I was agonized, and often attempted to rush to the window and to present myself to the mob and to save the lives of my friends, by my own sacrifice; at other times, to satisfy my curiosity, to see if my family and relations were really there. For, I had a species of doubts; but no one who has not been deranged, can understand how dreadfully true a lunatic's insane imagination appears to him, how slight his sane doubts. But I was not permitted to reach the window, and I was tied down again in bed; then my usual delusion came on me, that I was gifted with the power of an elephant to break my bands; and when I tried and found how futile were my efforts, I was told I did not choose to use the strength I had, from cowardice, or ingratitude, or laziness. On one occasion, I remember, after my brother had come to attend me, a spirit came to me whilst I was lying on my back, fatigued with my efforts to break the straight waistcoat, by forcing my arms and elbows out laterally, and said, *use my strength, I will show you how to do it*. The spirit then guided my arms and my hands, and with my fingers *sought and scratched the seams of the waistcoat sleeves*, soon loosened them, and I began tearing the seams asunder. The noise of the rending asunder however soon aroused my attendant, my straight waistcoat was taken off, and my arms were crossed over my stomach, in two heavy, hot, leathern arm pieces, which were not taken off from me for good, until I reached England. I feel thankful now for their removal.

CHAPTER X

THE DELUSIONS ABOVE DETAILED were accompanied with many other circumstances which I can hardly order aright in my memory; they were to this effect. That the angels and spirits of heaven from pity, and Satan and all his angels, being released from their torments, even by my sin, from gratitude and pity, combined to pray the Lord to suspend his judgments, to this end; that one only chance for my ultimate salvation might be given me. And this was, that by some signal act of obedience and acknowledgment of my divine mission, I might so purify my spirits and soul, before I suffered the punishments prepared for me on earth, and entered into my eternal judgments, that they, by uniting their spirits with mine, might enable me to endure them all, however cruel, in patience and obedience, so as ultimately to obtain my own pardon.

Although therefore my native genius, and the voice of one of my sister's spirits impelled me to sacrifice myself at any cost, and in any manner, rather than through my supineness or cowardice, cause the death and sufferings of so many defenders; yet another spirit, which I understood to be that of my Saviour, or of his immediate messenger, implored me not to do so, because, in so doing, *I must perish eternally*, and deprive him of the glory of making God's whole creation an universe of bliss.

It may be asked me, what course I would have had pursued towards me, seeing there was such evident danger in leaving me at liberty? I answer, that my conduct ought to have been tried in every situation compatible with my state; that I ought to have been dressed, if I would not dress myself; that I should have been invited to walk up and down my room, if not quietly, in the same confinement as in bed; that, whilst implements that might do me hurt were removed, pens, pencils, books, &c., should have been supplied to me; that I should have been placed in a hackney coach, and driven for air and exercise, towards the sea shore, and round the outskirts of Dublin. Few can imagine the sense of thirst and eager desire for freshness of air, which the recollection of that time yet excites in me. I do not recollect water having been presented to me, if it was, I systematically refused it, like every thing else; and it was not forced on me like the medicine and broth. If I recollect correctly, I got some water after my brother's arrival, and he also brought me once some grapes, a few of which I ate in spite of my false conscience, and God knows how refreshing they were.

To resume the thread of events; I felt a gradual relaxation of my muscular system, accompanied with a dreadful moral torpor and lethargy growing upon me, from my confinement and my regimen. It seemed to me at last as if humours rose up momentarily through the flesh of the face, which one by one stole from me the control of my muscles, and destroyed my moral energy. At the same time, I was accused by my spiritual tormentors of willing it, and it was *with* my will, though not *by* my will. I used to reply in inward deprecation, "I cannot help it, if I have no bracing exercise." I was then commanded to break my fetters, and told that I had strength given me to do so. I attempted it again and again; I was provoked to do it if only for exercise, but sunk as often, in hopeless indolence, and my feverishness and excitement were increased. Then, when I lay upon my pillow, a demand was made of me to suffocate myself on my pillow; that if I would do *that* in obedience to the Lord's Spirit, it would be an act of obedience, as grateful to him as any other I had been commanded. This delusion haunted me for many months. I imagined that I should be really suffocated, but saved from death, or raised from death, by miraculous interposition. I pressed my mouth and nostrils against the pillow; and I was to attend to the voices that came to me, directing my thoughts, and each tempting me to rise before I had executed the Lord's intention. I used to be deceived and to raise my head at some call, always out of time and place. I was accused of cowardice, and deceit. Night after night, and day after day, I was summoned to try it again and again till I should succeed, under the most awful penalties. I was told, that it was necessary for the perfection of the glorified man. That all the world had done it but me; that even my sisters had done it, that they had all done it repeatedly *for my sake, to put off my damnation*, because it was necessary that the commands of the Lord should be fulfilled when once spoken, and they hoped in time that I should do it by their aid. When I felt the chill of the outward air upon my neck under the bed clothes, I was told these were spirits of my sisters, breathing on me to cool me, and encouraging me to go through with my task. I was reminded that it was my only chance of salvation;

that, through my cowardice and want of fortitude, whole creations were suffering as yet the wrath of the Almighty, waiting for my obedience; and could not I, a man, do what women had done? At last, one hour, under an access[47] of chilling horror at my imagined loss of honour, I was unable to prevent the surrender of my judgment. The act of mind I describe, was accompanied with the sound of a slight crack, and the sensation of a fibre breaking over the right temple; it reminded me of the main-stay of a mast giving way; it was succeeded by a loss of control over certain of the muscles of my body, and was immediately followed by two other cracks of the same kind, one after the other, each more towards the right ear, followed by an additional relaxation of the muscles, and accompanied by an apparently additional surrender of the judgment. In fact, until now, I had retained a kind of restraining power over my thoughts and belief; I now had none; I could not resist the spiritual guilt and contamination of any thought, of any suggestion. My will to choose, to think orderly, was entirely gone, I became like one awake yet dreaming, present to the world in body, in spirit at the bar of heaven's judgment seat; or in hell, enduring terrors unutterable, by the preternatural menaces of everlasting and shocking torments; inexpressible anguish and remorse, from exaggerated accusations of my ingratitude, and a degrading and self-loathing sense of moral turpitude from accusations of crimes I had never committed. I had often conceived it probable that insanity was *occasioned by* a loss of honour; I had not suspected that an imagined loss of honour could also effect such a ruin.

The state of mind mentioned in the last chapter, was accompanied by many preternatural visions and experiences.

---

47   Onset, as of illness.

At one time, I saw the pale hand and arm of death stretched out over my bed. I felt no fear, but a sensation of confidence, that I was in God's keeping; if not for good, for evil. At another, I was desired to think orderly, and I was earnestly prayed to attempt it; but when I essayed, I was told I was doing nothing but "ruminate, ruminate all the day long." A moving light was given me, as a guide to know when I was ruminating or reflecting. It was a white light, and used to move in a circle from left to right upon the top of my bed. When I began to ruminate, it turned backwards to the left. Then my Saviour, or his angel's spirit, used to pray me to reflect, in order by any means to regain power over the muscles of my countenance. I say my Saviour or his angel, because when I imagined that I was in hell, that voice came to me, as the chief servant of Jesus in hell, directing and appointing the times and order of punishment and trial. I used also to hear a beautiful voice, that sung in the most tender, pure, and affecting notes these words, "Keep looking to Jesus, the author and finisher of thy salvation! Oh, keep looking—keep looking to Jesus!" Continually over the head of the bed, at the left-hand side, as if in the ceiling, *there was a sound as the voice of many waters,*[48] and I was made to imagine that the jets of gas, that came from the fire-place on the left-hand side, were the utterance of my Father's spirit, which was continually within me, attempting to save me, and continually obliged to return to be purified in hell fire, in consequence of the contamination it received from my foul thoughts. I make use of the language I heard. From the ceiling in front of my bed, I used to hear the decrees of what were called the assembly of counsellors, often ushered in these terms:

48 A phrase often used in the bible to describe the voice of God.

The will of Jehovah, the Lord is supreme—
He shall be obeyed, and thou must worship him!

The word of the Lord came from the left-hand side of the ceiling of the room, and many spirits assailed me from all quarters.

When I make use of these words, *ceiling of the room*, it will appear surprising, that the visions or sounds had such effect upon me, when sensible objects were present, and recognized by me. But I understood these things in a contrary sense. Besides in part seeing the white and flowing beards, and venerable countenances, I imagined I was really present to *them*; and that my not acknowledging it was a delusion, an obstinate resistance of the divine will on my part. That, of the two, the appearance of the bed, walls, and furniture, was false, *not* my preternatural impressions.

I had at times, in the course of my life, thought within myself on the doctrine of the *communion* of saints, the ubiquity and omniscience of God, and the power I attributed to the Deity of revealing thoughts and actions. The expressions in the Scripture of the church as a body resenting the sufferings of every member,[49] have led me to question whether, if we were in the spirit of God, we might not actually know and feel, each what the other was thinking about, or enduring, in various parts of the known world. That which had been a speculation, was now an act of faith; and I imagined that I could be in hell, on earth, and in heaven, at the same moment: nay, that I was, and that I witnessed all three states of existence; but that I did not see clearly the two extremes, because I would not acknowledge it to myself.

---

49 Corinthians 12:26: "And whether one member suffer, all the members suffer with it; or one member be honoured, all the members rejoice with it."

Indistinct ideas, also, of Bishop Berkeley's system, excepting against the reality of outward objects, from the experiences we have in dreams &c., helped this delusion.[50] For, reflecting on that system by the light of scripture, I put this question to myself, if the creation exists in my mind, under its present appearance, by the word of God, why may not my individual character, and the character of all objects now reflected on the mirror of the mind, be changed in a minute, and reiteratedly, by the word of the same God.

I was usually addressed in verse; and I was made to know that there were three degrees of hell; with the last of which among the worms, the moles, and the bats, I was often threatened. One day, when my head was towards the right hand corner of the bed, and I was lying on my back across it, with my feet tied to the left-hand bed-post at the bottom; I imagined I was being examined before the tribunal of the Almighty; an act of disobedience provoked the Almighty to cast me with a thunderbolt to hell, and the holy counsellors supplicated him to do so. An awful pause followed; I seemed removed to the gates of hell; and a stroke of lightning appeared to pierce the air on my right, but it did not strike me; for then the reason of my disobedience on earth, and the mystery of my sinfulness was revealed to me; and in a disconsolate and desolate state of mind, as one about to enter on a solitary and everlasting stage of suffering, I complained to myself that if I had but known these things before, and had I had but another trial allowed to me on earth, I hoped I might have done my duty. The voice I attributed to my Saviour recorded my

---

50   George Berkeley was an early eighteenth-century Irish philosopher who argued that matter exists through its perception in the mind—but that this perception was controlled by God.

thoughts aloud, as if he had staid by me to the last, and overheard me, saying, *he says so and so.* And I imagined it was agreed upon, that I should be tried again in this life upon earth.

On future occasions, I was often reminded of this engagement on my part, and I as often stipulated that the trial should not commence till I was restored to the state of health I enjoyed previously; but at the time, or on another day, when lying in the same position, I heard what resembled the notes of a hurdy-girdy,[51] which appeared to go round me, playing a tune that affected me with extreme anguish. It seemed to remind me of all that I had experienced and forgotten of my heavenly Father's care and love towards me. My mind, amidst other scenes, was transported back to Portugal—to a day when I had passed through Alhandra on horseback on my way to visit the lines of Torres Vedras, in company with three brother officers.[52] It appeared to me, as if that day a little Portuguese beggar boy had been playing on a hurdy-girdy in the street. But to my imagination, now, it was connected also with a time of life, when I had in person lived at Alhandra, a beggar orphan boy. When I had been taken charge of by the vicar or priest of the parish, who had loved me, clothed me, educated me, and provided for me as an assistant in the church. My protector had introduced me to the abbot of a monastery, and he also, a venerable old man, had been my patron. I rewarded them, by aiding in the robbery of the monastery chapel, with certain bad

51 A hurdy-gurdy is a stringed instrument played with a crank and a keyboard. It was popular in folk music.

52 The lines of Torres Vedras were a system of forts and walls built as the British and Portuguese defended Portugal from Napoleonic forces.

companions, and carrying off a golden relique, for the loss of which the old abbot had been sentenced to the flames by the Inquisition, being accused and condemned on presumption; and I had been too grossly sensual to come forward and save him. I had returned home, and in a few days I entered the sacristie, where was the vicar, and having assassinated him, stole his money and garments; which I disposed of and had fled to Cintra. The monks of Aldobaça had there met me, and I became for a time repentant; but I was taken into their convent, and became at last, with another lad, the servant and enjoyer of their unnatural lusts.[53]

During my residence there, I used often to visit Cintra, and in one farm house, being asked to assist in killing a pig, I had, to gratify my cruelty, plunged it alive into boiling water, after fastening up its mouth with sackcloth, to prevent its cries being heard.

This strange tale was revealed to me, accompanied with an impression of recollection, of identity with my own experience, as strongly as that by which any of the delusions of Pythagoras may have convinced him.[54] I remember I was first desired to recollect that portion of my life; and when I could not, the sounds of the hurdy-girdy were sent to me, as the voice said, to quicken my memory. I still had difficulty to collect any ideas, except my passing through Alhandra, my seeing the church on the right hand, and perhaps a young boy with a hurdy-girdy in the street or market-place. But an

---

53 Sintra and Aldobaça are towns in central Portugal, north of Lisbon. In describing monasteries as places of abuse and sin, Perceval was tapping into widespread anti-Catholic sentiment.

54 In addition to offering the Pythagorean theorem its name, Pythagoras believed in reincarnation, and believed that he had been a Trojan warrior in a past life.

indescribable sense of compunction, and of active interest in the place, wrung my feelings; and I was desired to recollect it as the place of my nativity.

I then heard a voice singing to the air of music

> I DO NOT REMEMBER THE HOUR AND THE DAY,
> BUT I DO REMEMBER THE DAY AND THE HOUR,
> WHEN I WAS A LITTLE BOY;*[55]

My difficulty of recollecting was charged on my wilfulness; and so I understood the two first lines, that I *would* not, not that I *could* not, remember, and this partly from compunction at the crimes I had committed on my patrons, partly from a sense of shame and guilt at the revelation of my acts of the monks of Aldobaça, which I imagined were being exposed in the presence of my fellow-countrymen, especially in that of the duke of Wellington, and the officers of my battalion; which also I was considered responsible for, although at the same time living in England in another body, in the discharge of my military duties.

When I inwardly expostulated and stated that when I was alive in England, I had not been aware of the union existing between me at the age of twenty-one, and a boy in Portugal of the age of seventeen; I was made to understand that an act of ingratitude in childhood had effaced from my mind the consciousness of this mystery, but that every individual besides me had experienced and delighted in this ubiquity of existence; and even that my brothers and sisters had been living in Portugal at the same time, and had

---

55   [Perceval's note] *"*I fear the death of my poor father was at the root of all my misfortunes; for I can trace the notes of this air, to the time we were living happily at Hampstead. I was then a little boy. But not now. I do not YET understand his loss."*

then been acquainted with me, and living in England, had been conscious of that acquaintance, but could not talk to me concerning it, by reason of my moral darkness through sin.

There was a horrid idea connected with this phrenzy, that in like manner as I had boiled the pig alive, I should be plunged into a huge copper of boiling water, and should be whirled round in it on my back with my mouth covered over with sackcloth, bubbling and boiling and drowning and suffocating for ever, and ever, and ever! My eyes were also to be taken out of my head, and I yet spiritually see them hanging over me, looking down upon me and pursuing me round the cauldron. To add to my horrors, my dearest friends would plunge me in and stand by ridiculing and tormenting me. I actually believed that a sound I heard in the room next to mine like to boiling water, was a preparation for this awful punishment, and that my brother and one of my cousins were every moment on the eve of plunging me in and condemning me for ever. When they came into my room I saw them at times like natural men, but at times their countenances appeared horridly swollen, and their faces darkened so that they looked black. Then I was told that I was not doing my duty to the Lord Jehovah supremely omnipotent, and that they appeared as the angels of hell, already prepared to execute the purposes of his wrath, but that I was always respited, in hope of my future obedience. My feelings were dreadful. On one of these occasions I recollect saying to my brother "—— I am desired to tell you you are a hypocrite." A voice had commanded me. This was one of the few sentences I addressed to any living being about me. I was commanded to say many things, but as the penalties were the same whether I did not say them, or used a wrong utterance, and I was constantly rebuked for the latter, and pained by a sense of ingratitude, I usually held my tongue, till urged by a new menace, or a new appeal, generally by the assurance that by the act of obedience, I should be redeeming thousands of souls who were suffering for me the agonies of hell fire, because I would not obey. Many times I called loudly after my brother and cousin, commanded to summon them and confess to them crimes of the most incredible nature. I recollect also, that I fancied myself to have been to blame for the drowning of an old woman, on the city side of the river, below Blackfriars bridge.[56]

I saw also visions of very heavenly forms in procession; and I was invited to come up to heavenly places; my inability was my crime. I also saw on my bed curtains, two, if not three faces, one of my Saviour, the other of my father, and of my Almighty Father; both white with long white beards. Once, after seeing the face representing my Almighty Father, I was accused of mocking, and I heard his voice saying severely and firmly, "I have sworn by my beard I will not be mocked at," which form of words were often repeated. A young man also who attended me, was named to me at one time as my fourth brother, at one time as my youngest brother; that he was so really, but that I would not acknowledge it to be so. But the vision which made the most vivid impression upon me, amounting to reality, so strong an impression indeed, that I might almost say, the possibility of being present in two places at the same time may be capable of realization; thine it was, O Lord, to interpret it to me. When I saw the venerable countenance of my father bending over me weeping, and the crystal tears falling, which I felt trickling down my shoulders, the impression of this was so vivid, that I can

---

56 The Blackfriars bridge spans the River Thames in London.

hardly help now suspecting, either that water was dropped on my back through the ceiling and tester of the bed, or that I was not where I appeared to be. Still it was not altogether the countenance of my father, as on earth; and I saw a long flowing white beard. I thought, could my father's beard have been so white and so long? But I both thought it unholy to question, and besides I could not control my thoughts to unravel my ideas. So my doubts took slight hold on my reason.

CHAPTER XI

BESIDES MY STRUGGLING to get loose from my manacles, and to reject the medicine and broth given me, I recollect only two active scenes. One day I was taken out at the right side of the bed, and held by men, whilst shaved on the crown. My friend Captain —— was in the room. I was desired by the Lord to be patient, till I saw his face at the window, and then to rise up and cry something. I did so. I saw the face; I rose up, and cried out, and then returned to bed. My chief grief at that time was, that I had received the tonsure of the Roman Catholic priesthood, a mark of the beast.[57] On another occasion when I was compelled to submit by force, and without the slightest word of explanation, to certain medical treatment, I was sensible of the indelicacy: on both, the option was given me to resist, and though I partially resisted, the fear of injury to my person *seems* to have biassed me to prefer submission.

When my brother first appeared by my bedside, "I have hopes now," said I, "I shall be understood and respected;" for

---

57   The tonsure is the shaved head of monk. Again, he associates Catholicism with evil.

he had written to me that he believed the reported miracles at Row.[58] When, however, I first told him, "I am desired to say so and so," "I am desired to do this, or that"—he replied to me, in an ill-judged tone of levity, and as if speaking to a child; ridiculing the idea. My hopes of being comprehended were blighted, and my heart turned from him. I reflected; my brother knew my powers of mind, he ought to consider that it can be no light matter that can so change me. I then resumed my silence, addressing no one except on a few occasions, and by command. Afterwards, as I got worse, I imagined the Almighty had cut short the times, and redeemed all men for my sins' sake, to visit all sins on my head; then I imagined also, that men now moved in a new life, knowing my thoughts and the Lord's thoughts, and the thoughts of one another. And when I was tempted to ask and ascertain any of these facts, I was told it was of no use, for that they would read whether I did so or not in obedience to the Lord, and, if I did not, would answer falsely.

Thus my delusions, or the meshes in which my reasoning faculties were entangled, became perfected; and it was next to impossible thoroughly to remove them, perhaps, for man's word alone, impossible.

Had my brother but said to himself, "there is something strange here; I will try to understand it"—had he but pretended to give credit to what I said, and reasoned with me on the matter revealed to me, acknowledging the possibility, but denying or questioning the divine nature of my inspirations; I should, perhaps, have been soon rescued from my dreadful situation, and saved from ruin: but it was not so.

---

58 His older brother Spencer would in fact later become an Apostle in the Irvingite movement.

During my confinement in Dublin, I knew no malice against any individual present with me, although I often contended with them. My mind was intensely occupied with the invisible agents I fancied to haunt me. Towards them I often indulged in spiteful acts of resistance and disobedience, overcome by the cruel taunts, and malevolent and contumelious language I received from them. At times, also, an inclination to humour or drollery made me dupe them—but this, more especially, a few months afterwards. These acts of disobedience were always combined with childish and absurd delusion. At one time, I took my medicine and swallowed it, with a design to poison the spirit residing in me: at another, I refused to suffocate myself on the pillow, to try to burst my manacles, or I drank my broth; in short, that conduct which people in their (so called) sound senses expected of me, I considered sin; that which they considered folly, I considered my duty; so completely was my judgment confounded.

Gradually I got better; I can hardly recollect how; but I remember a kind of confidence of mind came in me the evening after I had been threatened, and saw the thunderbolt fall harmless by my side, and when two days passed, and still found me safe in my bed. Also another night, shortly before I was removed from Dublin, I was trying to suffocate myself on the pillow as usual, when a command was given to one of my sisters to cut my throat, and my imagination was shocked by her accepting the office. Nothing ensuing, confidence again came in me, and this night a change took place in the tone of the voices. I recollect also a dream, in which I was in a bed in another house, during which I imagined that the Holy Ghost had descended upon me, like a downy cloud of a buff or nankeen colour,[59] and had sworn to bring me out of my troubles, and no more to forsake me. This dream left so strong an impression of reality, that it became the foundation of other delusions, but at the time it comforted me. However it was, I recollect I found myself one day left alone, and at liberty to leave my bed. I got up, and knelt down to pray. I did not pray, but I saw a vision, intended, as I understood, to convey to me the idea of the mechanism of the human mind! A morning or two after that, I was made to rise and dress, and left to breakfast; my brother breakfasted with me or after me; being desired by some spirits to leave the toast for him, a secret humour came upon me to eat it all up. I think I did so. It is to me still a mystery that I was so soon left alone for so long a time. Portmanteaus were being packed. I was made to go down stairs, get into a hackney coach, and go on board a Bristol packet. Whilst standing on the quay, I recognised a poor Irish lad, who used to hold my horse, and to do commissions for me; he had watched for me, and followed me, to see me embark. I could not express my feelings; but as he stood chill and shivering a little way off, there was an expression of distrust in his features; and I felt as if he were a truer friend than those occupied about my person.

---

59 Nankeen was a pale-yellow cotton cloth. Originally made from yellow cotton in Nanking, China, it was later made from regular cotton and dyed.

CHAPTER XII

WHEN I ENTERED THE PACKET, I descended with my brother and the stout servant who had hitherto attended me, into the cabin. I was desired to be seated; they attended to the portmanteaus. Unfortunately, either in obedience to the voices, or to my desire for action, I began walking about. In consequence, I was made to go to my bed, which God knows, I had had enough of. I soon became here again a sport of the wildest delusions. I imagined that on account of my sins, the ship and the whole ship's crew would be foundered on the voyage, unless I was thrown overboard like a second Jonah. I was desired to call out to my brother to come down; to inform him of the danger the ship was in; at one time to say one thing; at another, another; my brother came down; he put off my entreaties to let me come on deck; he joked at my fears. I then was desired to call for the captain. I called as loud as I could, but I was told it was not loud enough—that he had not heard me. That the storm was too loud—that I had, however, a voice given me, that would pierce through any confusion, but that my lethargy, my wilful, sinful lethargy,—alone prevented me using it.

I was then desired to prove that I was willing to sacrifice myself, and to overcome this lethargy, by getting out of my berth, and running upon deck. My servant struggled with me, and could only get me down by lying on me. This, of course, did not contribute to my health or comfort. At last, he got a pair of steel handcuffs on me. I was told it was my duty to slay him, that I might get on deck and devote myself to save the ship and crew. I struck at him with my manacled arms, endeavouring to kill him. When all my efforts availed nothing, I was still accused of lethargy and indifference, and made to consider this indifference the more dreadful, by the report that my dearest brothers, and many of my family who had come to Dublin to suffer and to die for me, were on deck likely to perish through my slothful ingratitude and stubborn refusal to make use of miraculous power given to me. At last, my servant got the leathern cases on my arms, and I was compelled to be the passive object of the tortures of my imagination.

The next morning we were moored alongside one of the quays at Bristol. When nearly all the passengers were on shore, I was conducted into the cabin; I recollect my brother being there and our standing by the stove; I think there was another gentleman there part of the time, and the captain came in soon after. I made some observations or answers, but I do not recollect what. My mind was recovering from the shock of its horrid delusions, and I felt a happy consciousness of my safety and of that of the crew, and a desire to realize it by being on shore. At the same time I felt an indignant hate towards the voices that had so acutely terrified me. But the next minute another snare was laid for me; that all that I saw around me was but a vision, that the ship had in reality foundered, and that the crew had been drowned, but that they, knowing the secret will of my Heavenly Father, and the dreadful and eternal torments prepared for me, had prayed to suffer death for me, whilst by the assistance of their spirits I was saved from the sense of the loss of the vessel and of my drowning until I could, by obtaining a repentant mind, undergo it hereafter patiently to my glory. However, my doubts were strong, and I now no longer obeyed the commands of these voices so implicitly. On landing, I called to my mind my landing near the same spot with my battalion in 1829. I accompanied my brother to an Hotel. I was shown up stairs into a large room with two beds in it. My brother remained with me. I was seated in an arm chair. A doctor entered, and with the sagacity belonging to the tribe, a sagacity by which they are sure to lose nothing, I was condemned again to my bed. I would have given my hand to remain up; my bed was a scene of horrors to me. However, I made no reply, and to bed I went.

I was scarcely in bed when I became a prey to new delusions. It was snowing at the time. I was told that a dreadful winter was to fall upon the country, on account of my sin. I was told that Bristol was on fire, and made to see flames; that the house was to fall and destroy every one in it; and this, all for my sin. My brother was sitting in the room with me. I expected every moment to see the walls crush him. I warned him to go away, for that the house was going to fall. I told him I saw the town in flames, he naturally made light of what I said. He recollected my words afterwards when the riots were in the town.[60] I was told that the reason he did not believe me was, that I did not address him in the tongue given to me; I was rebuked and upbraided for it. I essayed again, but I met with the same rebukes. I lost all patience.

---

60   The Bristol Riots of 1831. More on this later.

Again I was ordered to suffocate myself, and to kick about in various postures in the bed; unless I did so, that Satan would enter me, and that then my Saviour must endure in me fresh torments, to rescue my soul from hell. For though Satan was redeemed, yet he could only be my most skilful tormentor and destroyer, if I were not redeemed too, and delight also in his office, if I were at last reprobate. It seemed to me that Satan's spirit came to the left side of my bed and entered my body, and that I allowed it, for that I was so teazed that I delighted in the prospects of my Saviour's sufferings; immediately afterwards I was seized with compunction and dread.

The spirits also told me that a dinner would be brought to me; that some Irish stew had been ordered for me by my brother, which it was intended I should eat, but that a fowl would be sent me from heavenly places to tempt me, which I was to refuse. It was not the first time I had heard the like from the spirits, nor was it the last.

I did not understand what this meant, but I became very hungry. After some time the door opened, and a servant came in with the dish, containing a boiled fowl, which appeared very large and plump; I looked for the Irish stew, but it did not appear; the fowl on being brought near appeared small and meagre, and again plump, and twice its former size. The spirits then, to my inward observations, that there was but one dish, replied, that it was resolved to tempt me by a dish of the same kind, to make my trial more easy. That a fowl had been ordered for me on earth, as well as the fowl in heavenly places, because it was supposed I would at least consent to relinquish the second for the salvation of my soul, and the happiness of so many thousands interested in me; when I might eat the other. However the humour came upon me that I would dine in heavenly places as I called it, and I could not resist it; and yet it was *with* my will. For, after what I have related as having occurred in Dublin, I had no power to restrain my will, my cupidity, my avidity, from moral contamination, nay, the more I attempted to resist contamination, the more my power over my will seemed to evade me: besides this, there was a difficulty in obeying the commands given to me, because, even whilst eating the fowl, I was puzzled by the change in its appearance, and told, "now you must refuse it, because you are in heavenly places, now you may eat it because you are on earth, according as it appeared" beautiful or common.

The greater part of the night I passed in great torments. Next day I was in a post chaise with my brother on my road to Bath; the snow on the ground; in my mind earnestly desiring to be at home; and the voices dictating to me the conditions on which my Heavenly Father would allow my brother to take me home, and threatening other things if I did not perform these conditions. I was to utter certain phrases, make certain confessions, and the like. I thought I recollected the road along which I had marched in 1829, but I was not sure.

We turned to the left through some gates by a porter's lodge, a few miles on the road to London, and we drove up to a door of a house on the right hand side; we alighted, and I was ushered into a small room on the left hand side of the passage, and shortly after a young man came in, and then an old man, a very old man. I do not recollect being introduced to either. My brother went out and came in again. A man servant came and occupied himself in taking away the portmanteaus, and in laying the cloth for my dinner, he afterwards waited on me; He had a black coat on, and my spirits told me his name was Zachary Gibbs. All was in a mystery to me; only I understood that on certain conditions I was to go home, which *was all I desired* whilst on certain other conditions I was to be left here. The spirits told me this.

After the meat, a raspberry tartlet or two were brought to table; they appeared to be very large, clean, and beautiful, and I was told they were sent to me from heavenly places; that I was to refuse them; that they were sent to try me; that if I refused them I should be doing my duty, and my brother would take me to E——.[61] The same humour came on me to eat them all the quicker, under the idea that they had given me nothing but slops and physic for a fortnight or more, and now, if they are such fools as to bring me up into heavenly places, I'll make the best of it. My brother again went out, and I did not see him enter any more; this pained me exceedingly; I thought he would at least have bid me adieu; but the spirits told me that he was so disgusted at seeing me eating the tarts, when he knew that if I could only have refused one I should have been allowed by the Almighty to return to my mother and family, and that I knew it, that he had resolved to leave me without bidding adieu, and had given me up into the hands of the Almighty. I imagine now that his abrupt departure was preconcerted for fear of any opposition on my part.

Well, my brother went, and I was left amongst strangers.

If I had had any introduction to Dr. F. at least I was unconscious of it. I was left to account for my position in that asylum, for I was in Dr. F.'s asylum, to the working of my own, and be it recollected, a lunatic imagination?[62]

---

61   Ealing, the district in London where the Percevals lived.

62   Perceval has been placed in Brislington House (which he routinely spells "Brisslington"), an asylum outside of Bristol. Founded by Edward Long Fox,

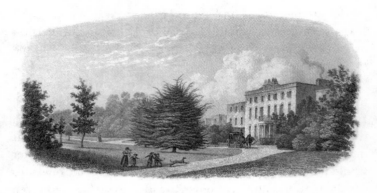

An etching of the asylum at Brislington as represented
in a promotional pamphlet printed by the Fox family.
Viewers will note an idyllic scene with dogs at play.

My spirits told me that I was in the house of an old
friend of my father's, where certain duties were expected of
me, that I knew what those duties were, but I pretended
ignorance because I was afraid of the malice and persecution
of the world in performing them. I persisted nevertheless in
inwardly maintaining my ignorance and in divining what
could be the meaning of these words. What ensued the evening my brother went away I do not recollect. I went to bed
in a small, narrow, disconsolate looking room with stuccoed
floor, over part of which was a carpet, bare white walls, a fire
place and fire in the corner, on the right hand side by the
window: the window opposite the door, the sill about the
height of a man's waist, white window blinds, a table, a wash-
hand-stand and a few chairs: on the left hand side, two beds,
occupying more than one third the breadth of the room, the

who remained on the premises, it was run at this time by two of his sons,
Francis and Charles. This was one of the most elite—and expensive—institutions in the country. For an extensive description of the asylum, see the
introduction to this volume.

one nearest the window with white bed hangings on a slight iron frame, the other nearer the door, made on the floor or very low: on this my attendant slept.

I was put to bed with my arms fastened. Either that night or the next, the heavy leathern cases were taken off my arms, to my great delight, and replaced by a straight waistcoat. The night brought to me my usual torments, but I slept during part of it sounder and better than before. In the morning I recollect observing a book of manuscript prayers, and a prayer book or bible bound in blue moroc-co;[63] the impression on my feelings was very dreary, and as if I had been imprisoned for a crime or for debt; but I was occupied as usual with the agony of mind occasioned by the incomprehensible commands, injunctions, insinuations, threats, taunts, insults, sarcasms, and pathetic appeals of the voices round me. Soon after I awoke, Zachary Gibbs made his appearance with a basin of tea and some bread and butter cut in small square pieces, about the size of those prepared for the holy sacrament. He staid in my room by my bed side, whilst I eat my breakfast.

I was not now aware that I was lunatic, nor did I admit this idea until the end of the year. I knew that I was pre-vented from discharging my duties to my Creator and to mankind, by some misunderstanding on my part; for which, on the authority of my spiritual accusers, I considered that I was wilfully guilty; racking my mind at the same time to divine their meaning. I imagined now that I was placed in this new position as a place of trial, that it might be seen whether I would persist in my malignant, or cowardly, or sluggish disobedience to the last. I imagined at the same time, that I was placed here *"to be taught of the spirits,"* that

---

63   A leather used for luxury book bindings.

is, (for they all spoke in different keys, tones, and measures, imitating usually the voices of relations or friends,) to learn what was the nature of each spirit that spoke to me, whether a spirit of fun, of humour, of sincerity, of honesty, of honour, of hypocrisy, of perfect obedience, or what not, and to acquire knowledge to answer to the suggestions or arguments of each, as they in turn addressed me, or to choose which I would obey.

For instance, whilst eating my breakfast, different spirits assailed me, trying me. One said, eat a piece of bread for my sake, &c., &c.; another at the same time would say, refuse it for my sake, or, refuse *that piece* for my sake and take *that*; others, in like manner, would direct me to take or refuse my tea. I could seldom refuse one, without disobeying the other; and to add to my disturbance of mind, at these unusual phenomena, and at the grief of mind—and at times alarm, I appeared to feel at disobeying any, Zachary Gibbs stood by my bed-side observing me in a new character. I understood that he was now no longer Zachary Gibbs, but a spiritual body called Herminet Herbert, the personification, in fact, of that spirit which had attended me in Dublin, so intimately united with my Saviour; indeed in my mind almost identified with Jesus.[64]

---

64 In the second edition of his memoir, Perceval would write: "Why I called this man Herminet Herbert I do not know, neither can I explain or define my understanding of the term, only I was told on my inquiring of my spirits the meaning of the words that I knew it very well, and I then endeavored to explain them thus with reference to the Greek and German languages—'Herminet'—the messenger, herald, or interpreter—'herr,' the Lord—'bert,' I could by no means translate, and the voices told me it meant 'of hell,' and I understood that Herminet Herbert was a familiar style by which souls under punishment might term the Lord, as a son calls his father 'governer,' or a debtor, his prison, his 'palace,' or 'castle.' I have found since, on referring to an old dictionary, that the word 'herbert,' or '*heer*-bert,' signifies Leader, or Lord of Hosts."

I understood that as a seal to the information I now received from my spirits, he had put on a nankeen jacket, in order by that colour to remind me of the dream, in which the Holy Ghost, who was his mother, had appeared to me, promising never to desert me. That he knew all my thoughts, and all I was inspired to do, and could not be deceived. He had come to aid me; but that at the same time, to prove my faith, that he would act as if he were a man in plain circumstances, if he saw I doubted.

Whilst therefore I was hesitating about each morsel I put into my mouth, he stood by, encouraging me to eat, and pressing me to finish my breakfast, or he would leave me and come back, saying, "What! have'nt you done yet?" Persuaded that he knew and commanded what was going on in my mind, I did not believe his encouragements sincere; but intended also to try me. I could not stand the ridicule I met with from my spirits, or to which I exposed myself in reality: I forced my conscience, wounding my spirits; teased, tormented, twitted, frightened, at times I was made to dupe my spirits by humor. Thus, it appeared to me that, whilst standing on the very threshold of heaven, eternal hell yawned at my feet; through my stupidity and impatience.

For about three mornings, my breakfast was brought to me in this manner; after breakfast, I was dressed, and for two or three days taken down to a small square parlour, with two windows opposite the entrance, looking over some leads into a court, thence over a garden to a flat country terminated by hills, about two or three miles off. The windows had iron Venetian blinds before them; looking through them, I saw snow on the leads; I was still under the impression that this was the effect of a dismal winter sent upon my country for my disobedience. There was a round mirror between the windows; in the left-hand side of the room, an iron fire-place with a fire in it. At the bottom of the grate, over the arch under which the cinders fall, a hideous face and mouth appeared moulded in the iron. At the end of the year, when I examined it again, I saw my eyes also had been deluded, unless the grate had been changed, for the ornament was a basket of flowers, not a face. Besides this, there was a horsehair sofa opposite the windows, against the wall; some chairs and a table; also a table against the wall in the centre of the room.

When I came into the room, there was a mild old rheumatic man there, who had on a white apron. He was of low stature, and in countenance resembling my father very strongly. My spirits informed me it was my father, who had been raised from the dead, in order, if possible, to assist in saving my soul. He was also in a spiritual body. Every thing in short, had been done to save me by quickening my affections, in order to overcome my torpor, and ingratitude, and fear of man. The chairs in the room, resembling those I had seen when a child in my father's dining-room; the very trees in the distance, resembling others in the prospect round my mother's house; almost all that I saw had been brought by the Almighty power, or infinite goodness of the Lord, and placed around me to quicken my feelings! If a man can imagine realizing these ideas, in any degree, awake, he may imagine what were my sufferings.

I asked now what I was to do. There was a newspaper lying on the table, but I could not read it, because, before I had been taken unwell in Dublin, when looking for guidance from the Holy Spirit, I had been diverted from reading the papers, except here and there, as if it were unwholesome to the mind. I thought it ungrateful now to have recourse to them for amusement, and for that reason, or "by that reply," in the language of my invisible companions, I decided my resolution, without quite satisfying them.

What was I to do? I was told it was necessary to do something "to keep my heart to my head, and my head to my heart," to prevent "my going into a wrong state of mind," phrases used to me. I was told, at length, to "waltz round the table, and see what I should see." I did that—nothing came of it. My attendant requested me to be quiet; at last, my dinner was brought. I had, if I recollect accurately, two dinners in this room—one was of a kind of forced meat;[65] the other had bacon with it: both meals were very light, and although I did not refuse them, I recollect feeling that I could have eaten something more substantial, and also being nauseated at the forced meat and bacon, which, I considered, could not be exactly wholesome for me.

My dinner in this room was served on a tray, with a napkin, silver forks, decanters, &c. &c., and in these respects, such as was fitting for a gentleman.

Unfortunately, the second day I think after my entrance into this asylum, having no books, no occupation, nothing to do but to look out of window, or read the newspaper, I was again excited by my spirits to waltz round the room; in doing this, or at a future period, I caught the reflection of my countenance in the mirror, I was shocked and stood still; my countenance looked round and unmeaning: I cried to myself, "Ichabod![66] my glory has departed from me," then I

---

65   Ground or pureed meat sometimes processed with herbs used as the stuffing for sausages, pates, and other molded meats.

66   Ichabod is an expression of lament or regret (something like a religious "Alas!"), in reference to 1 Samuel 4:21.

said to myself, what a hypocrite I look like! So far I was in a right state of mind; but the next thought was, "how shall I set about to destroy my hypocrisy;" then I became again lunatic. Then I resumed my waltzing, and being directed to do so, I took hold of my old attendant to waltz with him; but at last, deeming that absurd, and finding him refuse, the spirits said, "then wrestle with him if you will." I asked him to wrestle; he refused. I understood this was to try me if I was sincere; I seized him to force him to wrestle; he became alarmed; an old patient in the asylum passing by the door, hearing a struggle, entered, and assisted in putting me into a straight waistcoat: I was forced down on the sofa. He apologized to me for it many months after, saying it was in the afternoon, when all the other assistants were out walking with their respective patients.

Thus commenced my second ruin; and the history of an awful course of sufferings and cruelties, which terminated in my recovery from my delusions about the beginning of the next year, and was followed by my confinement as a madman, for nearly two years in a sound state of mind; because I entered into dispute with my family on their conduct to me, and the nature of my treatment, determined to bring them to account at law, for the warning of others, and to satisfy my excited sense of wrong.[67] I can no longer, after arriving at this period of my trials, call Dr. F——'s house by any other name than that it deserves, *mad-house*, for to call that, or any like that, an *asylum*, is cruel mockery and revolting duplicity!

I have already stated, that when I came to this house, I did not know that I was insane. And my insanity appears to

---

67 The difficulty of convincing others of your sanity when incarcerated in a madhouse formed much of the basis of Perceval's later advocacy with the Alleged Lunatics' Friend Society. He would discuss it at greater length in his second edition of this text.

me to have differed in one respect from that of many other patients; that I was not actuated by *impression* or feeling, but misled by audible inspiration, or *visible*, rather than *sensible* guidance of my limbs. To the voices I heard, and to these guidances, I surrendered up my judgment, or what remained to me of judgment, fearing that I should be disobeying the word of God, if I did not do so. When I first came to Dr. F—'s madhouse, my health was somewhat restored, my mind somewhat confirmed; yet my attendant informed me at the close of the year, I looked so ill when my brother left me, that he thought I could not live. I was like a child in thought and will, so far as my feelings were directed to those around me. I knew no malice, no vice. I imagined that they loved me, and were all deeply interested in the salvation of my soul, and I imagined too that I loved them dearly. Yet I wrestled with the keepers, and offered to do so with others, and struck many hard blows; sometimes, as one informed me, making it difficult for three strong men to control me, yet whenever I did this, I was commanded to do so. I was told that they knew I was commanded, that they wished me to do so, to prove my faith and courage, but that they were commanded to prove both till they were satisfied of my sincerity. I may safely say, that for nine entire months, if not for the whole of the period of my confinement in Dr. F —'s charge, I never spoke, hardly acted, and hardly thought, but by inspiration or guidance, and yet I suppose that never was there any one who so completely contradicted the will of the Almighty, or the desires of those around him, and I could not help laughing now at the delusions which made me constantly choose that conduct which was most disagreeable and terrifying to my doctor and his keepers, as in the reality the most agreeable to them, if I were not overcome by a sense of the cruel state of abandonment and exposure to their malice and ignorance in which I was left.

After being fastened in the straight waistcoat, I was taken down stairs to a long saloon or parlour, to the left of the little parlour I had been as yet confined to, and on the ground floor. There was a long table in the middle of the room, allowing space to pass round it, a fire on the left hand side, and a glass bow window and door at the further end. I was fastened in a niche on a painted wooden seat between the fire and the glass window, in the curve in the wall forming the bow at the end of the room; another niche opposite to me was occupied by a trembling grey headed old man; there were several other strange looking personages on the chairs about the room, and passing occasionally through the glass window door which looked out in the same direction as the windows of the room I had quitted, into a small court yard. I think I hear the door jarring now, as they slammed it to and fro. I marvelled at my position; my spirits told me that I was now in a mad-house, and I was told that it only remained for me to pray for the inmates, that they might be restored to their senses, and that they should be restored, but that I must then forego certain advantages. I attempted to pray, though I did not quite believe that I was in a mad-house, being unconscious of my own melancholy state, or imagining that I was placed there for convenience, not from necessity. There was an appearance of wretchedness and disorder amongst my associates, and I felt happy to be taken up to my bed-room after tea had been served in the evening.

The next morning my breakfast was brought to me as before in bed. I was dressed up stairs, and Herminet Herbert conducted me down to the seat I occupied the night before. There was an appearance of more cleanliness, order, and composure in the persons of the wretched individuals around me. Now I was told by my spirits that my prayer had been heard, that they had been restored to a sound state of mind, that they were in consequence among the redeemed of the Lord and knew that I had prayed for them, that they had in their turn desired to be allowed to remain with me one year as guides to me, and as a species of jury, to wait until I became obedient to the Almighty, and to judge me whether I was sincere in my difficulties or not; this delusion lasted for more than six months with this difference, that sometimes I conceived it my duty to recognize in their persons, relations, and friends, sometimes ministers and officers of the king.

The trembling grey headed old man was still opposite to me, and I was told that he was the Father Confessor, to whom I used to confess my sins in Portugal, and that he was there waiting to hear my confessions concerning my crimes as a poor lad at Alcobaça. Before my trials and punishments commenced, I was desired to confess to him. I tried several times, but I was checked by the noise, by his inattention, and by the rebukes of my spirits. He did not appear often after; whether he died or whether he was removed, I cannot say.

There were two or three volumes of a register in the room, and a large octavo bible.[68] I tried to read them but I was always puzzled and dodged by my tormentors, who could not let me rest, but made me turn from one place to another, usually guiding me after all to an anecdote about a Russian lady and a Czar of Russia, which I read over *till I was sick of it*, and which I perfectly understood. I recollect

---

68 The "register" here likely refers to volumes of a magazine or other compilation text. "Octavo" refers to the number of leaves that a printer would make by folding a full sheet of paper—here, eight. An octavo would usually not be a particularly large format in comparison to larger quarto or folio texts.

the first few days I was down in this room I was occasionally allowed to leave the niche in the evening, and sit by the fire or table, when I used to try to read these books; but one evening, Herminet Herbert on remarking my behaviour, for some cause fastened me up again; after that, I did not regain my liberty of action in doors for six or more months. It was in the cricketting season after the hay was made, that I was first allowed to walk about in the room and yard amongst my fellow prisoners.[69]

Not long after my introduction into this room, the three registers were taken away; the bible remained. When I was allowed to use my discretion, I used to read this in the yard, until an old lunatic, whom I imagined to be the Lord Jehovah, forbade me to do so, and I obeyed. I recollect the servant bringing it in soiled and defaced in the winter from under the privet hedge, where it had been hidden by one of the lunatics.

Besides this, occasionally one or two papers were brought into the room. My delusions increased so rapidly and became so confirmed after I was placed here, that my constant train of idea and habit of thought ran upon England, and this world, as of a creation gone by; I understood at one time that, the Almighty having cut short the times and redeemed the whole world, every part of the creation was changed, but that with a view to give me every chance of saving my soul, I was allowed to walk in a vision representing objects as they were when I was in England. I did not entirely believe these communications; still they had such an effect upon my mind that my form of thought was always "when I was in England," "when I was in the world."

---

69   According to later references, this would be around June.

I recollect with what eagerness I tried to get hold of the newspapers when I first saw them in this room, to discover if events were going on as I had left them, and what courage it gave me at first to read the articles of the war in Poland[70] accompanied with a comfortable assurance that I was still in the land of the living, like that related of one when he first saw a gibbet.[71] But now I was told that these papers were printed to try me, that the Almighty made me read just what he would, but that if I were redeemed I should see other words printed there, heavenly ideas which they who were around me saw.

I thought that the lapse of time had been concealed from me, and though really in hell one moment and in heaven another, yet I was only allowed to see around me events as they had taken place in England and elsewhere in the year 1831, after my illness in and removal from Dublin. That at that time the Almighty had caused the war in Poland to break out to atone for my sins, and had visited England with a destructive winter and pestilences on account of my blasphemies, and therefore now I read in the papers what had taken place as at that time.

For I imagined that whenever I disobeyed the word of the Lord or did not fulfil it, *pretending*, as I was accused of, not to understand it, the wrath of God commanded horrible torments on me, and that His word being once passed, it was necessary that they should be endured, and that I ultimately should myself suffer them: which I must either do in His power or in a state of rebellion and despair, wherefore

---

70 Likely the November Uprising, in which Polish forces rebelled against the Russian Empire in 1830-31. It was part of a larger wave of revolutionary movements across Europe at the time.

71 Gallows.

the spirits and persons round me and affected towards me, undertook to endure them as often as they were commanded, hoping for the time, that I should endure them to my own and to God's glory. But enough of these horrors and imbecilities for the present.

CHAPTER XIII

Let no man mock at the understanding; that could so patiently or humbly submit to such seemingly absurd teachings; but rather let him fear and pray that the power of the Lord to confound the judgment and wisdom of man may not be put forth upon him.

My mind was not destroyed, without the ruin of my body. My delusions, though they often made me ridiculous, did not derange my understanding unaided by the poisonous medicines and unnatural treatment of my physicians. Then when I became insane, the knowledge of that fact appears to have given to every one who had to deal with me carte blanche to act towards me, as far as seemed good unto himself, in defiance of nature, of common sense, and of humanity. The wonder is, not that I fell, but that, having through my fall come into the net which is spread by the arts and malice of the lunatic doctors, I could endure their treatment, and, recovering from under it, exercise my own native sense of justice boldly in spite of their will, whilst still unsound in judgment, and ultimately ride triumphant over the waves of misfortune! My senses were all mocked

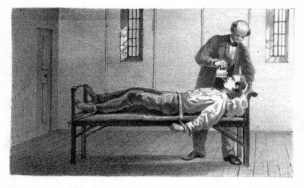

Ebenezer Haskell's 1869 asylum account included images of abusive
treatment. Here, he depicts a patient strapped down "in spread
eagle form": a treatment that he suggests could lead to death.

at and deceived. In reading, my eyes saw words in the paper
which when I looked again were not. The forms of those
around me and their features changed, even as I looked on
them. Nature appeared at times renewed, and in a beautiful
medium that reminded me of the promises of the gospel
and the prophecies concerning the times of refreshing and
renewal; in a few minutes she again appeared trite and barren
of virtue, as I had used to know her. I heard the voices of
invisible agents, and notes so divine, so pure, so holy, that
they alone perhaps might recompense me for my sufferings.
My sense of feeling was not the same, my smell, my taste,
gone or confounded.

Believing in miraculous agency, and the subject of
miraculous sensations, I received these as the word and
guidance of God, for their beauty and their apparent ten-
dency to promote purity and benevolence. And if I doubted,
my doubts were overwhelmed if not dissipated by compunction at attributing what was so kind, so lovely, so touching,

to any but the divine nature, and by fear of committing the sin against the Holy Ghost. Whatever then appeared contradictory, or did not turn out as I expected, I attributed to my disobedience or want of understanding, not to want of truth in my mediator.

CHAPTER XIV

THE NEXT MORNING after my entrance into the lunatics'
common room, I observed three men, apparently *servants*
or attendants of the gentlemen there. One was Herminet
Herbert, whom in a black coat I was to address as Zachary
Gibbs, and who I was afterwards told, on seeing him in a blue
coat, was Samuel Hobbs; but under all these appearances he
was one and the same Jesus. I used to call him Herminet
Herbert, the simple, and Jesus Christ. He was a short, active,
fair, witty, clever man. The other was a tall, spare, aquiline
nosed gawky man, from Devonshire, like a groom. The
voices told me to call him at times Herminet Herbert Scott,
at times, Sincerity; at times, Marshall; *that was his name.* The
third was a stout, jovial, powerful man, like a labourer. The
voices told me he was Herminet Herbert, the simple, God
Almighty, and that I was to call him SIMPLICITY; his name
was Poole. Besides this, a very stout, powerful dark man, like
a coach-man, with a very small voice and gentle manners,
was occasionally occupied in attending on me and other
patients. I called him by order Herminet Herbert the Holy
Ghost, or Kill-all. I understood these were incarnations or

manifestations of the Trinity. A stout benevolent old gentleman, a lunatic, who was dressed in a suit of blue, and
had been handsome, as I was informed, the Lord Jehovah,
supremely omnipotent, the trinity in unity, who had taken
upon himself the form of an old writing master who used
to teach me when a child, and whose name was Waldony,
by which name, and by that of Benevolence, I was at times
desired to address him. Likewise I understood Herminet
Herbert Scott, or Marshall, to be a favourite servant of my
Father's, who had lived in our family at Hampstead, and had
been raised from the dead with my father and my eldest sister to attend on me. And Herminet Herbert the simple, or
Samuel Hobbs, I was told had lived in my mother's family
after my father's death, and had been very fond of me and my
brothers, and familiar with us; that my brothers had known
at the time that he was Jesus, but that I had not; that during
an illness I had had when young, he had wrestled with me
in the school-room, it being necessary for my health, and
he had come now in hopes of winning me to wrestle with
him again, which was continually enjoined to me for the
salvation of my soul, and the keeping me in a right state of
mind. Several persons about the asylum, I was told, were
my father, Dr. F., a Dr. L., and two aged keepers, one of
whom I called Honesty; the other, my real father, because
he most resembled him. Now, when I did not recognize any
of these facts or any of these people, I was told it was on
account of my ingratitude and my cowardice. That I feared
to acknowledge objects as they were, because then I knew I
must prepare to endure my awful torments.

Now all these persons, and each person around me,
wore a triple character, according to each of which I was in
turns to address them. Samuel Hobbs, for example, was at

times to be worshipped in the character of Jesus, at times to be treated familiarly as Herminet Herbert, a spiritual body, at times to be dealt with as plain Samuel Hobbs. The stout old patient was at times knelt to as the Lord Jehovah; at times he was Mr. Waldony, a spiritual body; at times a gentleman. So with the rest: and these changes took place so instantaneously, that I was completely puzzled as to my deportment towards them. I saw individuals and members of the family of Dr. F——, approach me in great beauty, and in obedience to a voice, my inclinations sprang forward to salute them, when in an instant, their appearance changed, and another command made me hesitate and draw back. In the same manner, when books, pencils, pens, or any occupation was presented to me, I turned from one page and one object, to another, and back again, usually ending in a fit of exasperation and inward indignation, against the guidance that so perplexed me.

Besides the personages I have already taken notice of, there were eleven patients in the room, to each of which my spirits gave a name, and assigned a particular office towards me. There were three I addressed as Mr. Fitzherbert; a Captain P. who was my spirit of family pride; a Captain W——, who was my spirit of joviality; a Mr.——, a Quaker, who was my spirit of simplicity; a Mr. D————, who for a long time I imagined to be, and addressed as, Dr. F——, and afterwards as one of my uncles; a Mr. A——, who was my fifth brother, and my spirit of contrition; the Rev. Mr. J——, a Devonshire curate, who was one of my first cousins, my spirit of affection, and the representation of the apostle St. John; a Mr. J. who was my spirit of honesty, and my youngest brother; a Mr.——, who thought himself the Duke of Somerset, and whom I addressed as

Mr. Fazakerly,[72] my spirit of delicacy and contrition; and Captain —— ——a dark man, who had lost his left leg, and the use of his left arm; and who for six months stood up in one position, and for six months sat down in one position—him my spirits called patience; and told me he was my executioner, waiting for the decision of the jury upon me, to officiate on me, but still one of my best friends.

Besides these, the youngest Mrs. F—— —— was pointed out to me as repentance; two of the housekeepers as my mother, and two servant girls, one as a sister and a cousin, and one as my deceased sister. I was told that the reason I did not recognize them was, that I could not or would not, for sin. And certainly the countenances of those about changed in a wonderful manner. And I did at one time, amongst the patients see one of my aunts, who was many miles away; and on another occasion, I saw in a patient who was introduced into the common room in the summer, an old schoolfellow so like to him, that I called out his name in surprise; when the vision changed, and I saw him walking in other features, and then again in new ones.

In the midst of all this confusion of triple or quadruple persons in one and the same individual, and of my understanding, that according as my spirits warned me, I was either on earth as it was when I left it, or in heaven, or in an intermediate state of felicity, I was desired to act and to do my duty, and accused of guilt in pretending not to know what was my duty, and resisting the desire of the Lord to learn of my spirits. I might well be puzzled. I might well have been puzzled, setting aside that delusion. For it might be a trial for a very wise man to act discreetly on being ushered by violence or guile, into a room full of gentlemen who spoke

---

72 Fazakerly is a suburb of Liverpool.

nothing, did nothing, or muttered a few half sentences to him without being informed of the nature of his company and of his position amongst them. I had no introduction, no explanation, no reason assigned me for my position; lunatic, imbecile, childish, deluded, I was left to divine every thing. Precisely that conduct likeliest to aid deception of the mind, to encourage and to make it perpetual, was pursued towards me, and is now being pursued towards those wretched companions I have left behind me, and to tens of thousands in a similar state.

My earnest desire, my intense inward prayer to the Deity whom I imagined conversing in me, was, "Oh! take me home, Oh! take me to E——. I shall never know what I am to do here; all is so new, so strange, so perplexing. If I were one fortnight, one week, three days in the library at E——, left to myself, I should know how I was to act—what I was to do." My brothers, my sisters, and my mother were always in my thoughts; my constant longing was to be with them. Nearly all I did that was extravagant, nearly all the voluntary suffering I brought on myself was with a view to my finding myself miraculously amongst them, or them about me.

CHAPTER XV

A MORNING OR TWO after my removal to the lunatics' common room, I was dressed and taken down there to breakfast,
and this was continued until the beginning of the next year,
when I had recovered my sense enough to insist on treatment more becoming my wants, character, habits, and rank
in society. I came down with my attendant between half-
past six and half-past seven o'clock. The breakfast was usually placed on the table about eight. The tea was poured out
of two large beer cans into slop basons, and a plate of bread
and butter placed by each bason. There was seldom any
complaint from the patients, excepting poor Patience. He
always complained, in broken and rather violent sentences,
not addressed to any one particularly, of the thickness of
the slices. And I observed there was always placed on his
plate one slice, twice the thickness of all the rest. My spirits
assured me I was brought down stairs to show contempt
of me, and to punish me for my continued disobedience;
or for some particular act of rebellion in the eating of my
breakfast up stairs. I never made any remonstrance against
this or any treatment, however bad; so fully was I persuaded

that the persons around me acted from inspiration, and that my Saviour in Herminet Herbert directed every regulation, however severely, from necessity, and to my ultimate benefit.

Immediately on being brought down stairs, I was taken to my niche, seated down, and fastened into it by a strap with a small padlock, that ran through a ring in the wall, which ring could be turned round. My tea was placed before me, at breakfast time, in a slop basin, on a small deal table, with a plate of bread and butter. And usually one hand was loosened from the straight waistcoat; at times I was fed by the hand. It was always a great delight to me to get my hand at liberty, even for a moment, and the first use I usually made of it was to strike the keeper who untied me; directed by my spirits to do so, as the return he desired above all things else; because he knew I was proving my gratitude to the Lord Jehovah, at the risk of being struck myself. My blows were usually received in good humour. The same mysterious directions came to me at breakfast here, but my confusion was greater, and my humour to delude my spirits more strong. I disobeyed and deceived every voice; although told that I polluted my spirits by so doing. The voice which kept control over me the longest was that of my deceased sister, excepting only the voices of him whom I deemed the Lord Jehovah. At last, I disobeyed and mocked at even that voice; and then I became nearly reckless about obeying any or not; only being excited to try again and again to reconcile their directions by pathetic appeals, remonstrances, threats, awakenings of compunction and of remorse.

I disobeyed these voices, although at the time threatened with terrible consequences, and aware of the dreadful terrors of mind I should go through attended with accusations of impatience and ingratitude, when my meal was over,

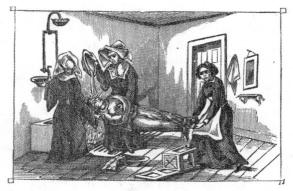

Forcible bathing as represented in Juliet Workman's 1877 exposé of the Mount Hope Retreat insane asylum. Workman's anti-Catholic sentiments and criticism of hydrotherapy will be familiar to Perceval's readers.

and my humour indulged. For instance, when a few weeks later they used to take me to the bath after breakfast, the spirits called to my mind their horrid threats in Dublin, and bade me understand, that this was the bath of boiling water, in which I was to be plunged for all eternity; I was threatened with finding it so, if I did not obey my spirits, or before I descended to it, reconcile them to me, by suffering something for their sakes. Two or three circumstances led to a confirmation of this delusion. In the first place, the bath was in gloomy rooms like cellars. In one room, in which I was usually dressed and undressed, there was no window at all, and the walls bare; in the other two, the light came from small windows at the top of the wall. We passed along passages to get to them, in which I saw large iron pipes, like the apparatus of steam-engines; and these I was told were to convey the hot water to the bath. I was occasionally seized hand and foot by two men, and thrown suddenly backwards into the bath: and I did not know what need there was for that violence, for I never hesitated to enter it. On one occasion, Simplicity stretched out an iron bar to duck my head under the water by pressing it upon my neck; for the men seemed to think it an essential part of their extraordinary quackery, to have the head well soused.[73] After ducking my head, he held the bar out to me in sport, and I seized hold of it, and found it quite warm, as if just taken from a fire. I attribute this now to the extreme coldness of my body in the water; for often, for half an hour after I came from the bath, I shook and shuddered, and my teeth chattered with cold; on these occasions I was usually fastened for a time alone in a large wicker chair, in the parlour I had originally been confined to. But at the time, I conceived the heat of the bar to be a proof to me accorded in mercy of what my spirits told me; that I was really in the bath of boiling water, concealed from me by their agency, but ready, on my provoking the Lord beyond redemption, to be instantaneously revealed to me. On another occasion, I entered the bath rooms after some other patients, when Herminet Herbert showed me a leather mask, which in sport he offered to put on me, and asked how I should like to go into the bath with it? Now my spirits had threatened me with being plunged in, after having my face covered with a pitch plaster. So these trifling incidents aided my delusions.

I may add here, that ere I had been plunged in the cold bath myself, which was not for at least a week after my arrival, I was threatened with it by my persecutors, and I used to see the patients called out one after the other, when my spirits always informed me, and indeed on any

---

73   Perceval is right: the Foxes put a great deal of faith in bathing, and they advertised that the asylum had a cold bath, a hot bath, a steam bath, and a shower.

extraordinary occasion, "Mr. Fitzherbert is gone for you—" or, "Mr. Simplicity is suffering for you." I was, in short, made accountable for every event around me, and continually appealed to, "will you suffer nothing for us, when we are suffering for you, in all those around you—things you ought to suffer?" I understood then that all these gentlemen went and endured the horrors of the bath of boiling water for me, rather than that I should undergo it in a state unable to endure it to God's glory and to my own salvation. My attendant came up to me one day, and said to me—some confusion having arisen—"you seem to be at the bottom of all that's going on here; what was it? you seem to understand all these things." On another day, when Herminet Herbert was going up stairs, and I was fastened in one of the niches, an old patient said to me, "there's your Saviour going up stairs; what! will you not go after him?" All these observations corroborated my delusions. I was told I had miraculous power to burst my manacles, but that I would not use it. One afternoon, when all were gone out walking, and I was left strapped up alone, my spirits told me power was given me to open my padlock, and be at liberty. I tried, and I did open the padlock, and was at liberty some time; till on their return, Herminet Herbert found me, and expressed his surprise, "How came you loose?" and locked me up again.

I may also add, that on one occasion, when I went to the bath, Herminet Herbert asked a man who was there—whom I afterwards, if I am not wrong, found out to be a bricklayer (one of the baths there appeared to be undergoing repairs)—to help him to throw me into the water. We had come downstairs alone. Usually, the hulking fellow I called the Holy Ghost, or Kill-all, came to my bedside, about half-past six in the morning, to help to take me down, for

I almost invariably resisted going down, not from my own notion, but by the command of my spirits, as doing the thing most agreeable to the attendants. I was told that this man was another personification of the Holy Ghost, and another Kill-all. For that as Diana was worshipped in two forms, as DIANA and HECATE, so the Holy Ghost was the destroyer of those in hell.[74] I saw this man, one day, in the passage, and his face was for a moment of a preternatural red or flame colour. He was at that time at work in a cellar opening in the front of the house, where I was made to believe that a cold bath was being prepared for me, into which I was to be plunged and immured in the dark; and to be always sinking and drowning to all eternity. I used to long to look down that cellar to see if it was true that preparations were really going on for a bath, but I never had an opportunity.

And there was, I must admit, also a singular coincidence between the state of mind, and trifling actions of those around, and the events that my spirits forewarned me of, or threatened me with, during the day. If, for instance, Mr. Fitzherbert, my spirit of family pride, who was pointed out to me as my guide came down with his shoes on, instead of looking for them in the room, or hung up his hat, my voices told me to augur such and such things during the day, which usually proved true.

---

74 Diana, the Roman version of the Greek Artemis, was worshipped by some as a tripartite Goddess: Diana, Luna, and Hecate. Hecate was associated with the underworld.

CHAPTER XVI

IN THE MORNING, after the breakfast things were removed, it was a natural thought to any mind to ask "what shall I do?" How to answer this, in a situation like that of the unfortunate gentlemen in that room whose limbs were at liberty, was difficult enough. There were three books, but what were they among so many? occasionally one or two newspapers, besides this a draft-board and a pack of cards. Soon after, the books were reduced to the bible, and then that disappeared.[75] But that which was a natural thought to others, was to me a question addressed to invisible guides, and rendered more difficult to answer, inasmuch as I was confined to my wooden seat, and often with my arms manacled. My voices first told me to speak to each Herminet Herbert as he came into the room. What was I to say? "Herminet Herbert, will you take me to my mother's room upstairs?" "Herminet Herbert, will you take me to my mother's room down stairs?" Though I shrunk from saying these things, yet I obeyed these voices. No attention

---

75 The Foxes advertised a robust system of activities, with a library, games, and outdoor recreation.

whatever was paid to me. I asked my spirits how my mother could have a room in that house? Afterwards two or three housekeepers in the mad-house were pointed out to me as my mother; I replied, I could not recognize her; I was answered, because I would not. I remarked how could she be so poor, and performing the offices of a menial? I was answered, that as part of the calamities and curses brought on my nation by the Almighty in consequence of my sins, a general bankruptcy had ruined the state and my family; that nevertheless the love of my family was such, that they had come to wait on me as servants of Dr. F., rather than abandon me. Poor things, they never came near me! How often did I struggle with my attendants, and provoke their violence to get to one or other of these rooms, imagining that my mother and sisters were waiting there to receive me, and that all that was required of me was to grapple with my antagonist, sincerely resolved to endure the extreme of his anger rather than shrink from doing what was enjoined on me. After I found that my addresses were of no avail, and I got tired of repeating the same words, I again asked for direction. I was desired then to address the old man opposite me, and to confess my sins in Portugal to him, as to my Father Confessor. I called to him, but received no reply; again I was directed to address the patients around me: another time to say, Herminet Herbert, will you take me to the w——— closet.[76] I suffered acutely in doing this, particularly before all the by-standers: but I yielded. After some time, I was attended to, and taken up stairs. Here I was usually conducted by him I called Simplicity, and God Almighty: I was assailed by new delusions. I used to rise from

---

76 Perceval has apparently abbreviated the phrase "water closet," or toilet, out of modesty.

the seat and throw myself forward, flat on my face, through the door, to fall at the feet of this individual and worship him. The door opened outwards, and I had my arms usually fastened round my waist. I therefore ran considerable risk of hurting myself, besides the punishment of this stout fellow. This extraordinary conduct was suggested to me in this manner. Although I was in the house of Dr. F. an old friend of my father's, upon earth, I was at the same time present in heavenly places: and capable of being conscious of both states of existence, and of directing my conduct in each, in rapidly succeeding intervals of time, according to what was passing round me in each. But the exercise of faith was required of me, and one great trial of that faith was to see the doors, walls, and persons round me as on earth. To cast myself prostrate before God Almighty in heavenly places was a reasonable act: to cast myself prostrate in a straight waistcoat, through the door of the closet, at the feet of a servant was not a reasonable act, and a dangerous one to boot. The apparent danger and reasonableness were the trial of my faith: and if I flung myself forward bodily, which through fear I seldom or ever succeeded in doing, exactly at the word of the Spirit sent to give me the time; I should find there was no door, no walls, no servant, no obstacle; but that I was verily in the presence of the saints, at the feet of Jehovah. I met, however, with nothing but severe falls and blows on my face and arms from the door, and rough handling from my attendant; who threw me back violently on the seat, and when there struck me in the abdomen, and then pitched into my face. My arms being tied, I used to turn my head to the right, and the blows fell on my left ear. This powerful man often struck me with great ferocity and spite: like one not contented with his situation, or perplexed by conduct unintelligible, which teazed him, whether designed or not. He was, however, generally good-humoured, and civil in his demeanour. Unfortunately, his punishment was of no use to me. I understood that I was punished for feigning, not for my act of faith, and the blows were another chance for my being at last miraculously at home, or in heavenly places. They only tended to disturb the equanimity of my mind in attempting to perform the duties required of me by my spiritual Mentors. Receiving their voices as the commands of my God, nothing could prevent me attempting to obey those commands, however absurd they might appear to myself or others, or dangerous to myself. The awful impression of dread produced by preternatural menaces; the compunction I felt for former acts of ingratitude; the appeals to my attachment, sense of honour, sense of duty, made by my spirits; the hope of redeeming millions of souls by one act of obedience, and of standing in the presence of Jesus and his Father, were too strong for me to resist. Experience alone of the falsehood of the promises could succeed in making me relinquish altogether my attempt; and that experience was long in coming, for fear or embarrassment continually made me prevent or lag behind the instant of execution; and then the failure of effect was attributed to my not acting with "precision and decision."

Returning to the common room, I always attempted to wrestle with, or asked one of the patients to wrestle with me, I was then locked into my seat. If my arms were at liberty, I would occasionally seize one or two of the patients to wrestle with me as they passed by me. I had no malicious motive; I did it in obedience to inspiration, and imagined they were inspired to know what I was commanded, how

I obeyed, and how to act in consequence. My attempts at wrestling were however inculcated by the spirits on more practical grounds than ordinary. They told me that it was necessary "for the *keeping me in a right state of mind*," in other words, "to keep my head to my heart, and my heart to my head;" that I should be suffocated, or strangled, or violently exercised, or at least perform one act of obedience to the Lord Jehovah supremely Omnipotent, in a certain rhyme or measure once or twice through the day; that without that my head wandered from my heart, and my heart turned from my head all through the day, which was the cause of my being in a wrong state of mind; by which expression I did not then understand lunacy. I used to ask several individuals to wrestle with me, with a view to their giving me violent usage, a severe fall and the like, and with the secret hope that during the wrestling, one or other of them would strangle me or cause me to suffocate. I always seized the strongest men, and it is a singular fact, whilst I compelled the other keepers to struggle with me, I never did more than lay hold of the waistcoat of him I called Jesus, the weakest, unless when I was struggling with three at a time. The men usually held my arms, joked with me, begged me to be quiet, and used no more violence than was requisite to overcome me. Therefore I did not get what I wanted, until the autumn, when one day seizing Sincerity to wrestle with him, he gave me a tremendous fall that shook my whole frame. I knew then I had done my duty, and finding myself no more in heavenly places than I was at the beginning, not a whit more capable of understanding my position, I desisted from any further attempts of that kind.

But before I received this fall I was made to fancy that my insincerity prevented the man from dealing with me as

God intended; that they knew I was shuffling; that I did not exert half the force I had; yet at the end of the year Samuel Poole reminded me saying, "how you used to make us sweat!" for three keepers usually came to compel me to go to the cold bath, which to me was a mystery, because I was not aware force was required to take me there, and I was told I might go to the bath with Simplicity, or Sincerity, or Herminet Herbert, according to my conduct. But in reality it was, I conclude, a display of force to intimidate; in which it failed through my delusions, for it provoked my efforts. But it answered another purpose, that my foolish opposition did not meet with such cruel violence as the spite or fears of a weaker party might have inflicted on me. Sometimes I was carried along in sport neck and crop; but usually I did not meet, on these occasions, except from single hands, with ruder treatment than might be expected from three country fellows overcoming resistance: on one occasion only I recollect a stick being brought out to beat me, but I do not recollect its being used. I am not sure.

When consigned to my seat, it became again a question how I was to employ myself. I felt in this position a sense of suffocation, which together with former delusions, suggested to me the idea of suffocating myself by pressing my nostrils against a wooden projection in the wall serving as an arm to the seat. This in fact was my chief occupation all the day long, occasionally varied by my attempting to twist my neck, standing up as well as I could and leaning on the back of my head, the face turned upwards against the wall, and then turning my body as on a pivot from side to side. Occasionally an old patient put a newspaper on my knees to read, and Herminet Herbert once or twice gave me one of the registers. Sometimes my hands were untied for a short

time to read them. In the morning, and always in the afternoon, certain of the patients smoked and sat down with the
servants to a game at whist.[77] Scarcely a word was spoken
except in broken sentences, or by the servants, which added
to the apparent mystery of my situation. Once a day usually,
one or more of Dr. F.'s sons came into the room and staid
five or ten minutes, he addressed one or two patients, and
occasionally said a few words to me; but always with a half
and half manner of speech and deportment, which added to
the conviction I was under, that they too came for a mysterious purpose. Occasionally they smoked a cigar in the room,
and played a game at cards. I was told that one of these
gentlemen was my brother D., and his name Sincerity and
Contrition; the other, my brother H., and his name Joviality;
he was an amiable good-looking fellow; the other, melancholy, and besotted. I occasionally asked these and other
well dressed men to wrestle with me, but I did not attempt
to force them, in spite of my spirits, for they were too well
dressed, too decent, too childish. Generally every Sunday
morning about ten o'clock, Dr. F., the father of these young
men, tottered in, a grey-headed firm-charactered old man,
of short stature, with a blue frock coat on, broad brimmed
hat, and long cane. But to me all was delusion; I thought him
a spiritual being; I called him my father.

About 11 o'clock every day, the patients were taken out
walking, if the weather was fine, and I went out for an hour
with Herminet Herbert, or was left tied up alone. Dinner
came at one; in the afternoon the patients again went out
for a walk, came home about four, went into the yard or
sat down in the room till seven, when tea was brought and
served as the breakfast; after which, they were taken or

77 A card game.

went alone upstairs to bed.[78] Besides this, during the day
they were occasionally taken out one by one, either to the
bath or to be shaved, but I then understood when they went
out singly, they went either to suffer, or to supplicate for me;
when they went out together, they went as a court of justice
to consult on my case.

When I was first fastened in my niche, my feet were at
liberty, but afterwards they also were fastened by leathern
sockets to a ring in the floor. There were two or three reasons for this, or rather causes; for had my treatment been
reasonable there would I conceive have been little reason
for any personal confinement at all. I imagine now that I
was unwittingly the servant of a spirit employed to mock at
all the conceits of a presumptuous charlatan and his careless servants, for controlling, overcoming, or managing the
human mind; which spirit did at the same time work to my
punishment and degradation. When I was fastened down,
for example, in the niche with my hands secured round my
waist and my body girt with a leathern belt to the wall, my
spirits guided me to turn completely round heels over head,
so that my neck came against the seat, my feet reached the
arch of the niche, and, raised up on one side, came down on
the other. It is astonishing I never hurt myself. They cut off
this strange amusement by fastening my feet to the floor. I
used also after dinner and breakfast to kick over the table
with the plate at times on it, and when my feet were fastened
I used to lean down and do this with my mouth; sometimes
I succeeded, sometimes I did not, but my aim was to do it in
"*precision and decision*," and I did not care how many blows I
received, though I feared them, if they would give me only

---

78   A regular schedule was a hallmark of the "moral treatment" offered in
asylums like Dr. Fox's.

three *in precision and decision*. I was often struck, but usually only two blows at a time; Simplicity struck me most. At last, towards the end of six months, I got three blows and three sharp raps from a spoon, from Herminet Herbert, in the time or measure I conceived was required, and finding myself still in the same situation in mind and body, I did not attempt any thing, merely to seek their blows, any longer. I used also to try and drag things to me with my feet, sometimes to fling my shoes off into the room, &c. &c., and I would actually wait in silent faith and prayer for the shoe to come back to me.

This was my position in this room for about three months; after that, I was removed to the niche in the wall opposite to the fire-place, and continued confined there till late in the cricketting season, after hay making.[79]

About three days after I was left by my brother, I was taken out for my first walk by Herminet Herbert. The snow-drop was just piercing the ground, and from that I judged afterwards I had been brought there towards the middle of January, for I had no means of calculating time, but by the seasons, and when by chance I got a newspaper; until in the autumn, coming to my senses, I asked for a pocket-book. I walked about Dr. F.'s grounds and plantations, crying out at every carriage I saw, that it was my mother's; to every young female that she was one of my sisters, and calling aloud by inspiration, "I am the lost hope of a noble family—I am ruined! I'm ruined! I'm lost! I'm undone! but I AM the redeemed of the Lord; I AM the redeemed of the Lord Jehovah supremely omnipotent, and of the Lord Jehovah Gireth, and of the Lord Jehovah, &c. &c. &c. who is

---

79   If the cricketing season began in June as earlier noted, this would suggest later in the summer.

true to his word, and his saints love it well;" *which last words also came to me in Dublin.*

The above sentences were given to me to repeat, laying a stress on the word "am," of which sentences I now see the beauty and the connexion, though then I cried each out separately, timidly, and undecidedly. The keeper who attended me occasionally rebuked me, ridiculed me, shook me, or struck me with his walking stick. Very often we walked out in the fields, and to farm-houses in the neighbourhood, when I used to fall down on my knees before this man, and call him Jesus. I had on, generally, a great coat over a straight waistcoat; so that at any moment my arms might be fastened. I walked usually for one hour before dinner, sometimes for an hour after dinner. After some time, I accompanied the other patients, who walked out in a body, with two or three keepers, and we went through the villages: here, as before, I cried out aloud, though not so often; and I did not desist from this for a long time. I recollect on one occasion, I ran away in the grounds from the keeper, who had desired me to keep by his side. He caught me by an iron fence in the grounds, and with great violence doubled me over it. On another occasion, looking up into the sky, I saw a vision of the Lord descending with the angels and saints. Several times, the sounds of the cattle lowing, or asses braying, in the fields, conveyed to me articulate words and sentences, as to Balaam.[80] I was often made a joke of in good humour by the keepers, on account of my delusions, and this added

---

80   A prophet in Numbers 22-24. When Balaam's donkey sees an angel it turns aside. Each time, Balaam beats the ass for disobeying him. Finally, God speaks through the animal: "What have I done unto thee, that thou hast smitten me these three times?...*Am* not I thine ass, upon which thou hast ridden ever since *I was* thine unto this day? was I ever wont to do so unto thee?" (Numbers 22: 28, 30).

to their strength, for I took seriously what they said in jest. For instance, one said to me, "there's your father, go and run after him, and take him by his arm," pointing to a patient I took for my father; another, whom I called Scott, but whose name was Marshall, replied one day, "*I am called Scott in good company*;" another walking behind my back, with an open knife, pricked me slightly on the shoulder-blade: I then had the most horrible ideas that I was to be crucified in a number of bodies in all parts of the world, to be flayed alive, &c. &c., and imagined that my doom was put off only from day to day: each time I came home to dinner I fancied was the last. This slight action of the keeper confirmed me in my horrid suspicions. Another delusion I laboured under was, that I should keep my head and heart together, and so serve the Lord, by throwing myself head over heels over every stile or gate I came to; the condition here was as before, on its being done *in precision and decision*. I often attempted and failed, getting smart strokes from the cane of Herminet Herbert. I knew it was dangerous, but I expected to be miraculously preserved if I did it aright. At last I did it outright, and my head struck upon a stone, on the other side. The blow stupified me: finding no advantage, I did not attempt it heartily again. On returning home, I was fastened in the niche, and remained there till bed-time.

Nobody can bear this continual turning of the mind from one subject to another; but I am not able to collect my ideas on these sufferings, so as to write orderly. I should add that I received the blows of Herminet Herbert patiently and without reply; first, being too much occupied by the agonies of my mind; secondly, conceiving that he was acting a part which he was compelled to do, to punish my insincerity and affectation; for that I was struck, not for attempting, but because I did not accomplish the object of throwing myself over the stile—through disobedience. I mention such delusions, as appear to me necessary to make my reader clearly understand the nature of my disorder, the state of my mind and disposition which I was in, and the impropriety of the conduct pursued towards me. To this end it appears I must still mention two other delusions connected one with the other. Soon after my arrival from Bristol I was told, by my invisible companions, that I was not the son of my reputed mother, but that my father had adopted me from my infancy. That my real name was Robinson. That my father and mother were Americans, from Boston. That my father had died long ago, but that my real mother, Mrs. Robinson, was still living at Bristol. I had known this until about eight or nine years of age, and my reputed father had adopted me, because he knew very well, I was ordained to be a herald of the second coming of the Lord, from my conception. And as the Almighty, in the shape of Mr. Waldong, had always walked on earth with my reputed father, in love, in gratitude, and in obedience to him, he had adopted me. I, too, had known this, until by one crime at an early age, my heart had been turned from God; after which, I had walked in darkness. At the same time, I had resolved to deny my father and mother, and would not allow any person to allude to the fact of my adoption. My reason and judgment checked me in believing this strange tale, but I bowed my reason to the authority of the inspiration!

I was told that when I passed through Bristol, I had been specially brought there to be tried if compunction would then make me call for my mother, Dame Robinson; and that she had even entered my room, in hopes of being reconciled. That had I shown even *that* gratitude towards her and towards the Almighty, I should have been spared many torments; but that when my countrymen saw I was so ungrateful, they had prayed for and determined on an increase of my tortures. I was already to be crucified for my blasphemies in Dublin, but now I was to be crucified, and "licked, and hacked, and manacled, and brewed in a manner most distressing" all over the world, in various bodies, and kept alive during my tortures. I objected, that the king of England could only hang me, but I was replied to, "that the king and parliament had passed an act for my especial punishment, in obedience to the commands of the Almighty, when he had come upon the earth." I imagined at one time, that my eldest sister, who had been raised from the dead, had undertaken to endure these tortures for me. Sometimes I fancied she was being flayed alive in the room downstairs, to which I strove to make my way; sometimes that she was being mangled in the garden, outside our prison room; and I used to strain my neck from my seat to look through the window to ascertain the truth. About this time, also, a packet was lost off the Welsh coast, and all the passengers were drowned. Much talking there was about it, and I was made in my imagination responsible for their loss; all was done for me. At night and by day I heard their groans; and on one occasion, when I understood I had done an act of obedience, there was a burst of angel voices, in the ceiling on the left, singing out, "Victoria, Victoria! the victory's won." I knew about as much what victory was alluded to, as what sins I was accused of.

I recollect, a short time before the burning of the gaols in Bristol,[81] in a letter I wrote to my mother, I asked her if

---

81 The 1831 Bristol riots were part of a pro-democracy movement. Very few in Bristol had the right to vote, and parliamentary representation was corrupt.

I was really her son, and if I had ever had a master called Waldong. I was then gradually returning to my senses. My mother sent me a certificate of my baptism, in Lincoln's Inn fields,[82] and shortly after, one of my brothers saw me, and reminded me of the real name of our writing-master when boys, and confirmed the suspicions I then had of my having been deluded. My mind, however, needed these circumstantial evidences, to be corrected entirely of its errors.

When a magistrate who was instrumental in rejecting a reform bill visited Bristol, locals rioted. The tone of the riots led some in government to fear that the nation would see a revolution like the one in France.

82   A park in London.

CHAPTER XVII

WHEN I WAS TAKEN to bed at first, I was only confined in my straight waistcoat. The first night there was a fire in my room, which I missed the second or third night, and I was made to suppose I had been deprived of it for not performing some act of obedience. A few nights after my arrival, I threw myself off the bed, in my waistcoat on the floor, in obedience to my monitors; the command was usually given about the time the keeper came into the room either to look after me, or to sleep; fortunately I did not injure my limbs. In consequence of this trick, my arms were tied down to each side of the bed, by bands of ticking. Still I contrived to excite alarm, and subsequently my feet were fastened to the bottom of the bed, in the leathern anklets I had on in the day time. Fastened thus, lying on my back, I passed my wretched sleepless nights for nearly, if not quite, nine months! Recollect, too, that I was a *nervous* patient! I had not exercise enough during the day to procure sleep, but I lay exhausted, wearied, agonied, terrified in my spirits, hungering after rest, but unable to procure it. To add to my feverishness and misery, the servant usually tied my

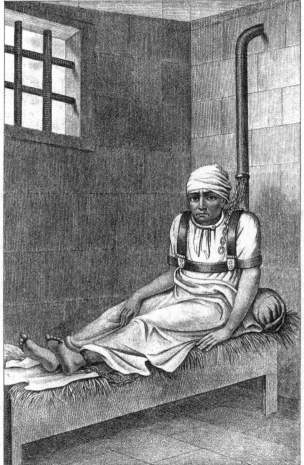

A patient chained to their bed in Bedlam from
Esquirol's *Des maladies mentales*.

right arm so tight, passing the thong twice round it, that it cut my flesh, causing a red ring round the arm in the morning.

I never complained; the voices told me it was Jesus who did it, and that he did it for my good, to prevent me going to sleep, because sleep would torpify me, and as I was a spiritual body, I did not need sleep. Sometimes, however, by order of the voices, I asked the servant when he came to bed to undo my right arm; which was occasionally done. In the coldest nights I used to kick off, or throw off with my teeth the clothes, yet I never felt cold.

This restraint was kept on a great while longer than was necessary. A lunatic doctor, in one sense, is pretty sure to be on the right side; he will run no risk that will do his reputation for security, an injury. When I began to come to my senses, and to feel indignation at the treatment I had been exposed to, the voices and my wishes dictated to me to ask to have the waistcoat taken off in bed, and I fancied one day, that I was invited to make this demand by young Dr. F. who stopped me, and the keeper, Samuel Hobbs, on going out of the madhouse to walk, asking if I could not be allowed to sleep unfastened now. The keeper replied, in an offhand impertinent manner, "O! no, sir—there's no trusting him," &c. &c. &c., and I remained silent from resentment.

After I was in bed, from about eight to ten o'clock, when the keeper came up, I very often used to shout out aloud, or sing the psalm, "O be joyful," in obedience to the demon's commands. Then Simplicity would come up, and with his open hand strike me on the face most cruelly—all I could do, tied hand and foot, was to turn my face to the wall, to avoid being struck in the eye, or on the nose. His blows fell on my left ear, as below stairs, and to these blows I attribute the disfigurement of my left ear, which afterwards swelled to a great size with extravasated blood. It was cut open by the surgeon who attended the patients in the asylum, Dr. L—. It is true, Dr. F. told my mother it was occasioned by violence I did my own person, in striking my ear, but I do not recollect striking my ear, but I recollect very well I used to strike the side of my head in front of the ear, where the organ of secrecy is placed, under an idea that my blows would strike out the secrets of my conscience and memory to me;[83] and after my ear became bad, and particularly after the operation, I tried by squeezing it against the wall, to burst the blood out, which was called "breaking my ear to my father." I imagined also, that the blood in my ear was caused by the lachrymatory duct[84] being full of tears of blood, which I would not weep; and other absurdities.

---

83 Perceval is referring to popular beliefs about phrenology, which held that the brain was made up of several "organs," or regions responsible for various mental activities and personality traits, like "hope," "conscientiousness," "bibativeness" (propensity to drink), "calculation," and "individuality." One's personality could thus be read by measuring the shape of one's skull.

84 Tear-duct.

CHAPTER XVIII

THERE WERE, HOWEVER, other serious inconveniences attendant upon my confinement in bed, of which I fear I now
feel the effects: viz:[85] the retention of my urine. My honest
doctor never thought of that, no doubt. I cannot express
myself becomingly on matters of this kind. My excited feelings prompt me to use expressions of sarcasm and indignation: but again, ridicule overpowers me for I say—why? why?
remonstrate upon any one isolated act, when the whole system, admitted by, and finding society fellow-workers with it,
is grossly disgraceful to men of science, to men of education,
to men of humanity, to men of religion, contradictory even
of the principles of that tangible science, surgery; not to say
medicine, of which Dr. F. and many more too like him, are
professors and practitioners! *But such men, surgeons,—and yet
acting inhumanly in defiance even of that sure science*, ought to
know that it is no small duty of the curer of nervous patients,
to have regard to the regularity of their evacuations. And
there is no point for which they more require what liberty
can be granted them. There is a moment, beyond which the

---

85 A shortening of *videlicet*: "namely," or "that is to say."

retention of urine becomes very deleterious to the circulating fluids, and affects the nervous system with acute pains. I knew nothing of this then; I have observed it subsequently. For the agonies of my mind were too great for me to heed bodily suffering.

Connected with this subject, I have to relate conduct towards me of the most indelicate and insulting nature. I do not recollect during the first months of my confinement any attention to me in this particular, volunteered on the part of those whose duty it was to think for me. I myself first asked to be taken upstairs, in obedience to inspiration. My mind has always been extremely sensitive and delicate on this subject, and it was with much difficulty and dislike that I obeyed the command given to me, in the presence of the other patients. After my daily visit to this place, I do not recollect any opportunity being offered me of discharging my urine, during the day, so long as I was confined to my seat, except in the morning, when I went out walking, and if I went out in the afternoon; but I do not remember that I made use of these opportunities. Sometimes, indeed, I refused to follow nature, understanding that being no longer a natural but a spiritual body, these things were no longer necessary, but on the contrary, injurious to me.

It happened however towards June, or July, that I was unable to contain my urine whilst in bed two mornings successively, overcome by fear whilst waiting for my keepers, who came to take me to the cold bath in reality, but as I imagined to my eternal doom. I used to lie in agony of fear, crying out to my different spiritual companions, "Herminet Herbert come to my room and save me from my melancholy doom and destiny." "Mr. Simplicity come to my room, &c. &c.," "Kill-all, Kill-all, come to my room, &c., &c.;" and I

used to augur for my fate according to who presented himself. I recollect now a sensation of fear, a sense of cruelty
which I cannot yet define as the men came up stairs and
entered my room to untie me. Their footsteps talked to me
as they came upstairs, the breathing of their nostrils over me
as they unfastened me, whispered threatenings; a machine I
used to hear at work pumping, spoke horrors; besides this,
there were some ducks and chickens came to be fed before
the window; a breakfast bell rung, and I heard a piano down
stairs: all these circumstances reminded me forcibly of my
boyhood, and I think my mind was afflicted with speechless
agony, at the comparison of my actual state with that of my
infancy, childhood, and youth; to have been so loved, or so
duped by the appearance of my family's love, and to be so
abandoned in the greatest woe, under the most awful state
of misfortune. But I accused myself of all, and chiefly for
bringing discredit upon the new doctrines of the Rowites,
on my own sincerity as a professor of religion, &c., thereby
endangering the salvation of those dearest me, by alienating
their affections from, and shaking to their confidence in, the
truth. The dinner bell used to ring to me many changes.
"This is Mr.———'s dinner bell at E———, if he will be obedient to a spirit of precision and decision, or, if he *will* do his
duty and not have his greed taken away from him," or "take
the young hypocrite to his mother's bed-room at E———, or
to his sister's schoolroom at E———, &c."

To return, one or two mornings whilst listening to all
these preternatural intimidations, and misinterpreting
them, my fears or my necessity compelled me to make water
in my bed. A night or two after this I was taken down to
sleep in a kind of outhouse. At the back of Dr. F.'s mad-
house at the bottom of all the small yards or gardens that lay

on the slope of the hill behind the different wards, a range of low buildings extended along the whole of that side of the mansion excepting the laundry. These buildings contained in each ward, three or four cells with bare walls, lighted by a small skylight from the top, with a channelled and sloping wooden frame for a bed, furnished with straps, chains, &c. I imagined this to be an instrument of torture. There was a narrow dark passage between the cells and the yard, and they were built against Dr. F.'s kitchen garden wall, which was warmed by flues. The kitchen garden lay behind the mad-house; the hot-houses[86] nearly in the centre. There was a small yard at the end of the four cells in our section with a door leading into the kitchen garden, and in the right hand corner near that door a privy.[87]

I was taken to bed in the innermost cell, the fourth in the row. There was a mattrass of straw, and a pillow of straw, both stinking of the cowyard, on which I was laid. I was then strapped down with a broad strap over my chest, and my right arm was manacled to a chain in the wall. No explanation of any kind was made to me, and I was left alone to my own meditations.

For myself, I submitted to every thing with passive resignation, and like a child. I conceived myself in circumstances hopelessly beyond my control; the object of the direct and personal superintendance of the Almighty. I did not understand, and it was useless to remonstrate; but my attendant voices suggested to me two or three reasons for my being thus degraded; either because I had eaten my breakfast instead of refusing it; or had not struck or wrestled with my keepers, or thrown them into the bath, when ordered to do

86 Bathhouses.
87 Outdoor toilet.

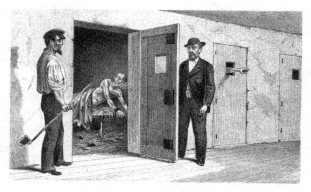

Haskell portrays the particularly dire situation at the rural Somerset County Madhouse, where patients were kept in dungeon-like cells.

so. The real reason was never clearly assigned to me, but I conjecture it was the design to punish me for the infirmity I have just alluded to; a design as foolish as it was insolent and unjust. Foolish, because no explanation was given to me, no expostulation, and I was left a lunatic to my lunatic imagination to supply me with a reason, if I reasoned at all. Foolish, because even if an explanation had been offered, it is doubtful then if I should have believed that, instead of the wild suggestions of my inspirers; therefore foolish and cruel, because as a correction it was of no use; and had I had strength of mind just sufficient to understand it as a correction, ten to one that I should have resented it by repeating the offence fifty times, rather than not show my hatred and contempt of their malice. Insolent it was, because no man has a right in a matter of this kind to deal thus with his equal or even with a child, far less a set of ignorant empirics and their tools.[88] Degraded it is true by a signal calamity, but yet

---

88 "Empiric" was a term for a medical practitioner who operated based on

their superior in rank and education, and entitled to respect even for the greatness of his misfortune, and to forbearance, for his infirmities. Unjust it was, for it was not marvellous that I had been twice subject to this inability of retention, but rather a marvel that I had not already *often* been so subject from their neglect.

About two or three hours after my being put to bed here, one of the keepers, Herminet Herbert the simple, or Herminet Herbert, Simplicity, came to attend to my bodily requirements in this respect, and then left me for the night.

Strange as it may appear, I felt happy in this situation. Here there was comparative peace, seclusion, freedom from intrusion. Here I had no servant sleeping in the room with me. Here I might hollo or sing as my spirits commanded, without fear of rating and beating, and although my right arm was fastened by a short chain to the wall and the strap pressed rather tightly across my chest, it was still something to have one arm free even in the straight waistcoat, and not to be galled by the fastening on the other. At first I tried as usual to suffocate myself in the pillow, the smell of which reminded me of a cow yard; but when I was weary of attempting what I could not perform, I turned my head round and lay completely on my back, looking up to the skylight, and wildly ruminating.

The sides of the skylight were partly open, for it was a bell light. It was apparently a fine night, but whether it rained or not was the same to me. I saw a star or two pass over me, and I saw a light that moved round in the heavens, and I was told it was the light that had appeared to the wise men or shepherds in the East, and that it had been sent

---

observation rather than medical theory. It was often used in a derogatory sense, implying a lack of formal training.

to comfort me. The rattling or rather grating of the chain against the wall, spoke to me in my father's voice. I was in the cell about a fortnight. The second night the straw pillow was removed, and a white plume pillow put in its place.

There are a few humane hearts that will shudder and shrink at the view of this position, recollecting my birth, my education, my talents, and that I had not been an impious or irreflecting man. But they will say it was the fault of the doctor, and though they condemn the doctor, still it was but the doctor. But no, oh! no, my elder brother came to visit me at this very time. I might almost say he seemed guided by providence to detect the cruel infamies of my situation. But he came and inspected the cell in which I was confined at night, he saw me and took leave of me in the evening sitting in my straight waistcoat in the niche, exposed to my fellow patients, and he left me to my fate. So great, so rooted are this world's hypocrisies, so deep and wide spreading its duplicity! so weak are so called sane man's imbecilities; imbecilities, such as make me less ashamed of having been a mad-man, when I think of the disgrace of such conduct, of such credulity, lightness, and triviality, unaccompanied and unexcused by disease.

In about a fortnight I was removed back to sleep in my former apartment. After that the keeper came to my bed side, regularly once each night, and without untying me, administered to my necessities, whilst I turned round on my left side as far as I could, performing for me, to my utter disgust, the most indelicate and revolting offices.

At the end of the year when I was awakened from my dream and lethargy, I inquired of Samuel Hobbs and Marshall, the reason of my having been placed in the cells; I received a kind of half answer from Hobbs, that it was on account of my infirmity in bed, to which Marshall added an observation, that he had remarked to his fellow servants, that he thought it a pity I had not more liberty in bed, as he conceived I must suffer at times from the long retention.

I have observed I used at my own desire to be taken at first to a closet upstairs. Here I often counteracted the desire of nature. Whether I did so or not, no more attention was paid to me on that score during the day. After some time I was taken to a place in the yard, or to that I have mentioned in the small court by the cells. In this latter I was placed on a seat in which I was fastened by a wooden bar in front, and by a manacle to my right hand, and there I was left, I dare say for half an hour at a time; and there I heard many voices and saw many phantasms.

In this same place in the summer time, when the water failed in the cold bath, which was often but dirty, I was made to undergo a kind of shower-bath. I was undressed in one of the cells, and accompanied by the two servants, walked naked across the little court to the "*cloaca*,"[89] on which I was seated and fastened in; Hobbs and the other then went and fetched two or three pails or cans of water. There were two brackets in the corner of this place over the seat on the right and left, on which Hobbs then mounted astride over me. He took one of the pails with him and with a pewter urinal ladled the contents of it over me, or poured it gradually out of the beer can. The shock used to convulse me a great deal, and besides I used to hold back my head with my mouth open and hallooing or panting, by which I was often nearly choked with the quantity of water that came down my throat. When the water was expended I was taken off the seat not without attempting to kneel or throw myself on my

---

89 Another term for the outdoor bathroom.

face before the men, who I conceived were spiritual bodies, or Jesus, or God Almighty; then I was dressed and reseated in my niche till the hour of exercise or till dinner time.

Other painful instances of neglect in the matters alluded to in this chapter, to which the other patients and I were subjected, I pass over.

CHAPTER XIX

MY TOILETTE[90] was very much neglected, and served as an occasion for insult and gross treatment on many occasions. At first after being taken to the bath I was brought up in the morning to my room to wash my hands and my teeth. But when I began either to throw myself on the floor or to turn round and round in the room whilst the keeper was making my bed, or even when I did not set directly to work, he would take the toothbrush violently from me, and either wash my hands or fasten my straight waistcoat round me without washing me, and take me down stairs. In general the plunge in the cold bath was considered dressing enough, sometimes I had not even that, but being taken down stairs unwashed, the bowl which served to wash the tea things was brought with clean water, and I was washed in my niche before the other patients and rubbed dry with a coarse duster, an insult to them as well as to me. My feet were not washed the whole time I was imbecile. The first time I attempted to judge for myself was to ask leave not to go to the cold

90 Habits of cleanliness, such as washing, shaving, dressing, or doing one's hair.

bath in the autumn, I felt as if soaked with water, it was granted. The second was to ask for water to wash my feet, the request surprised my servant; it was given me with some demur. They were begrimed. The toe nails had never been cut, and I had lost the nail of my little toe. My finger nails were cut by Herminet Herbert regularly, and always as low as they could be, as if to disfigure them. Two or three towels were brought to my room a week, but whether or no for my own use alone I do not know. There was for a long time no glass in my room. Once a week Herminet Herbert (Hobbs) brought my linen to my room which lay on a chair, three or four shirts and as many pairs of stockings. I had about two pocket handkerchiefs a week, sometimes none. The clothes I walked about the country in I was quite ashamed of, or rather I thought I ought to be ashamed of when I came to myself. When my eldest brother came to see me, I recollect I was taken into a room near the sitting room and dressed like a school-boy in a new suit previous to my being ushered into the parlour. I was then taken quite by surprise, and knew not what to expect.

It is my suspicion that a great deal of this treatment was designed to insult, under the idea of quickening, arousing, nettling the patient's feelings! but there is so much of evident neglect in the management, and so much may be the natural consequence of a system calculated on the strictest economy, and whereby the case of a gentleman is left almost to the entire control of a set of ignorant, simple, at times malevolent, and perhaps not over-honest servants, that it is not possible for me to determine; and besides, my mind is astonished at the idea of reasonable beings admitting the propriety of such gross mockery, arguing in so absurd a circle, to such a cruel end. It is as if when a jaded post horse has fallen motionless from fatigue you were to seek out a raw place to spur him or lash him in, to make him show symptoms of life. Again I say to myself, if this treatment was intended to insult, why was my indignation at it when I came to my senses condemned as madness? For so it was, which ever way it is, whether the doctors are simple agents of that destroying spirit, that works in their patients rendering them their victims, or whether they act designedly, the system is a cruel mockery of the patient. He is professedly a pitiable object of scrupulous care, the innocent dupe of unintelligible delusion, but he is treated as if responsible, as if his dupery is his fault; yet if he resists the treatment he is then a madman! and if, as in my case, he is agonized and downcast by a continual and unmeasured self-accusation of his great guilt in being insane, he receives no correcting intimation that he has something to say for himself, that he is the appalling witness of the power of disease; no encouragement, no inspiration of self-confidence; but all around tends to keep down his spirits, to depress his energies, to abase and degrade him in his own estimation. A short time before I left the mad-house, a Captain W., an officer in the army, complained to me one morning, evidently deeply perplexed, saying he had asked several times for a clean pocket handkerchief, and the one in his pocket he had had three days. He attributed it to the regulations of the laundry, but then, said he, they allow us I am told three a week, and I ought to have one. I told him I imagined that it was designed to insult him, and that I thought he would admit as much if he considered other parts of the system, and I added they shall not get me to ask them for any thing. I advised him to write to his father, and I wrote to my family *commanding* them to attend to my reasonable desires; they had the folly and wickedness to deny me or to defer justice.

If the insulting and degrading treatment I have described, was indeed designed to mortify and probe the feelings, it was preposterous, without explanation, expostulation, or remonstrance; and impolitic, without a thorough knowledge of the temper and humour of the individual to whom it was applied. Why was I confined? because I was a lunatic. And what is a lunatic, but one whose reasoning cannot be depended upon; one of imperfect and deranged understanding, and of a diseased imagination? What, then, was the natural consequence of my being placed in the most extraordinary, difficult, and unreasonable circumstances, without explanation, but that I should, as I did, attribute that insult which was heaped upon me to the most absurd causes; to the non-performance of the very acts, which in a sane mind I might have condemned; or to the performance of those which I might have applauded. With me, conscience was entirely confounded—judgment perverted. That which others called sin, I deemed virtue; that which men call folly, I called wisdom. What can be said, when I struck, kicked, wrestled, endangered my own security and that of others, as the acts most pleasing to them to witness, most dutiful for me to attempt? The reader now, perhaps, wonders at treatment like this being possible; but if he does now resent it, in nine cases out of ten it is not without my having been obliged to reason with him as with a child; so rooted is the prejudice, *that lunacy cannot be subdued, except by harsh treatment*. If he asks why these things are so, I will tell him why: *because it is the interest of the lunatic doctors*. That is the end. And the cause lies in the servile folly of mankind, of which these lunatic doctors make their profit.

But such treatment is impolitic, not in the lunatic doctor, but in the conduct of such as, in good faith, desire a patient's cure; because, if discovered or suspected, it may work, as it did in me, a deadly hate towards those dealing with me, and a resolution to endure any thing, rather than bow a haughty and stubborn spirit to their cunning, address, or cruelty, in return for their insolent severity, the mind mocks at their care and vigilance, their respect and their benevolence. The question, then, lies between the power of the patient to endure, and the power of the quack to break his spirit. The latter is shamefully uncontrolled by law, in consequence of the very generous, legitimate, and simple confidence placed by chancellors, magistrates, and law-officers of the crown in the humane, and tender, and scrupulous doctor. I have proved that the power of the patient is equal to that of the oppressor. But in this contest, when the patience and fortitude of the first is exhausted, look to it if the stamina of the constitution—if those foundations of sound health, are not undermined or broken through, on which, with respectful and natural treatment, cure, *perfect cure*, might have been established, and good citizens assured to the state; not those patched-up pieces of work called healed patients, now returned to the world. And again, besides the danger thus incurred, through the sullen and obstinate resentment of the patient, I have proved how, through his very disease, through his very delusions, the power of the spirit of evil mocks at such endeavours to subdue his empire over our conduct and our imaginations, without the will of the individual working malignantly with him.

Mine was not a solitary instance. Another patient in that madhouse, who, I observed, seldom or never spoke,— when one was hinting to me, that he thought the servants were directed to insult and degrade us, or, at least, did it designedly, of their own malevolence,—opened his lips, to my astonishment, and declared that when he first came to the asylum, whilst sitting one evening in the parlour wherein we were, he rang the bell, or called for a candle for another gentleman, when the servant came up, and, grossly insulting him, turned him, too, out of the room, and sent him to bed; since which, says he, I have never opened my mouth, except when absolutely necessary. Upon my pressing for further information, he resumed his silence; and though his conduct did not appear to me extremely wise, yet I can tell gentlemen who condemn it, that though it is a very comfortable doctrine for the lunatic doctors, and for a set of indolent and inefficient magistrates, to doubt and deny credit to a lunatic gentleman's word, we understand their insolence, and feel their injustice, though we cannot express our opinions, and dare not retaliate. And we beg leave to differ in our opinion. The only resource for the pride of many men is in a stubborn silence, and outward indifference. It is not surprising, then, if that is the only resource of the lunatic; of whom, it appears, all possible moral perfections are to be expected, instead of allowance being made for all possible moral weakness, whilst he is cut off from all human aid.

To return to the article of toilette. I was shaved three times a-week: Saturday was one of those days. Occasionally I was taken up to my own bed-room for this operation; but usually, for one half the year, I was ushered in, in turn with the other gentlemen, to a small room belonging to another, I fancy to old Patience, on the same floor with our common room; and the rest of the year, to a small servant's bed-room up stairs. In this room, there was one patient tying his neckcloth, another sitting to be shaved, and a third pulling off his coat; besides two servants and occasionally three. After being shaved, I was washed in the dirty water the rest had been using, and rubbed dry with the servant's dirty towel; and then, with a slight shove on the back, told to go down again to the sitting-room; or else I walked down arm in arm with Herminet Herbert, as I imagined my Saviour. I used at first repeatedly to ask the barber to cut my throat, in obedience to voices I heard; but I did not want it. I was always very nervous when being shaved, and found my mind more disturbed by it than at any other time, when I began to know my situation. It was also one of the circumstances that touched me with most sorrow and indignation, when I came to myself. For as a military man, I had always shaved every day; and I thought, if my friends had been disposed to show me any delicate attention during my illness, it would have been to have kept up my ancient military habits. But it is ridiculous to talk of delicacy. I recollect, also, when recovering, that one of the first shocks I felt my mind received, was in turning accidentally to the glass in the door of a dark closet, where the knives were cleaned, and seeing that my whiskers were cut short. I had never touched them from a lad, and used to take pleasure in their curls. I observed, on catching my face in the pane of glass, that my head involuntarily glanced away; and I turned back, to reflect what had struck me. I then recollected the day Marshall had cut my hair, in a chair at the end of the yard; and his manner had appeared to me very starch and sarcastic. I cannot say whether it was done for insult, or according to his idea of beauty. But it was disrespectful; for they might leave their patients, at least, as they find them, in such respects. The insult was either at the time thrown away upon me, or, as I think, my mind too much overwhelmed by my calamity and by my situation to notice it.

When I began to be more trusted, I was invited to dine in the afternoon with the young Dr. F. and his pretty little wife. I called her Repentance. Two or three patients usually dined with them at one time. Herminet Herbert waited on us, and a beautiful servant-girl, whom I called Louisa, and believed to be my sister. I contrived to get through the dinner without any very extraordinary actions or expressions, and afterwards I used to dine occasionally in the old doctor's mansion, in greater company; and though yet in a dream, my behaviour there was still more moderate. My spirits directed my attention with great rapidity to the objects of furniture, books, curtains, pillars, glasses, &c., in the room, and to little acts of civility. And I attribute my better manners to the greater occupation given to my imagination by variety of situation and ornament, and to my being in circumstances more congenial to my habits, and sensible of the impression of decent conduct and formalities around me.

I was much amused, about the middle of summer, when I was more collected, at the style of invitation sent to me. The old housekeeper came in, and said, "You *are to send* Mr. P. and two other patients in to dine with young Dr. F." I heard this accidentally; usually, I knew nothing of the great favour intended till the hour came, or by not being fed at the common table. When I heard the message, I was at first amused; then I thought, Do they intend to insult me? or is it the servant's fault? and my spirits dictated to me to be high-minded, and not to go. But I replied. Pooh! children! they don't care for me, and I don't care for them; let them alone!

On these occasions, Herminet Herbert took me up stairs to wash my hands, or brought down a clean white cravat, and a clean pair of shoes to put on, before I entered the ladies' presence. But one day, one of these attentions was neglected, after I had asked for it; or for another reason, perhaps because I was not shaved. I determined to refuse dining with them, not thinking myself fit to appear in the ladies' society. But the opinion or will of the patient was not once thought of in this matter: to refuse was in vain. I was pushed on, partly in humour, partly in earnest, by Herminet Herbert; and just as I was going to fight him, Mrs. F. and her husband issued from the drawing-room; and out of respect to her I ceased, and went to dinner.

I was taken down to the bath generally in the morning, but occasionally in the forenoon. In the morning, a great-coat or dressing-gown was thrown over me, and I went up stairs again to dress. Often, however, I was dressed in the cells adjoining the baths, by one or two keepers. Here I used to be directed to dodge my feet about, to untie what they had fastened, to throw off what they put on, to rise up from my chair, and to wrestle with them. There was a bath repairing in one of the cells, into which I was often prompted to throw Herminet Herbert backward; but although I was told it was what he desired, I could not conquer my fear of its causing his death. On one occasion, I was alone in the cell with this man, when he was putting on my stockings; and I bent forward, as usual, to prevent him: he threw me backward with great violence against the wall, and my head came with such force against the bricks, that a light seemed to strike through it, and I was almost stupified. But such acts were not extraordinary.

I now come to an important part of the regulations of this madhouse; the mockery of sending us to church, so it was called. A large room at the end of the building, which in week days served as a laundry, was on Sunday converted into a chapel. The female patients sat in the further end, with Dr. F.'s family, separated from the male by a screen. Would any sensible people believe it possible that I was taken, in my state of mind, to assist at this service? I went there believing that I was about to attend a kind of condemned sermon each time, after which, I was to be plunged into the bath, in which I was to be drowning for ever, and ever, and ever, for not having performed one act of duty to the Lord Jehovah supremely omnipotent; for not having struck properly, or wrestled properly, with one of the keepers. But I had a chance offered me of escaping my melancholy doom, if I would get up and wrestle with one of the keepers present. Sure enough up I got, and sometimes seized Simplicity, sometimes Sincerity; who then hurried me away crying out aloud. There was attention shown to me however, in this instance, that Dr. F. F. came and sat beside me, persuading me to be quiet.[91] This room was paved with square flagstones, and when in my mind I objected to wrestling in it, because it was paved with stone, I looked again, and saw it was regularly boarded, but it was really in stone. It was these miracles of the imagination made me cling to the delusion of being in two or three places at once.

After several experiments, I was left alone on Sunday evening in the sitting room, with the old gentleman I called Jehovah Gireth, who, fortunately for him, was a Roman Catholic; and so enjoyed that evening an hour's peace. But

---

91 Brislington House being a family establishment, the anonymized Doctors Fox become difficult to differentiate. Dr. F.F. refers to Francis Ker Fox. Francis and his brother, Charles, ran the asylum upon the retirement of its founder, their father Edward Long Fox. Perceval's later references to "Old Dr. Fox" are likely to Edward. It is less clear which Fox is intended by "Dr. F." alone.

when I began to recover my intellect, I was taken to this sad exhibition, this congregation of demons as I called them, again. I found, however, that my feelings were too acutely excited by the liturgy and the recollections the service awakened, for me to command them; and that, unless I wished to expose myself more disagreeably, my only chance was to turn things to ridicule. I was laughing, therefore, the whole service through, and, fearing that that in the end would harden my heart, I applied for leave to abstain from church. This was granted; but subsequently, when I had struck one of my keepers on a Saturday, either of his own private spite, or by order of Dr. F. *as a punishment, I was desired to attend church next evening.* I refused, and was offended; but recollecting myself, I took up my hat, and walked on in silence, seating myself in the church until Dr. F. F. came in. I was determined then not to submit to their cursed rule any longer, but to assert my own rights, and I rose up to meet him, and told him it was my desire not to attend the church service. He tried to silence me, but I persisted; and he then said aloud and contemptuously, "Take Mr. P. out; I must not let him disturb the congregation." Simplicity took me out, and as he lumbered after me, he tapped me with the key of the room on my shoulder, deprecating my conduct, and saying good-humoredly, "Come, come, Mr. P. no more of this; we shall be obliged to put you in a straight waistcoat again." He thought that I was returning to insanity because I resisted the doctor; or else he knew that the opposition of lunatics returning to reason, was so met; but I was confident in my powers of mind, and resolved to dispute usurped authority.

Now for the medical care taken of me. I was called in courtesy, and I was in the truest sense, a nervous patient.

Through disease, through medicine, through fever, and through mental anxiety. I was brought to Dr. F. immediately. The first diet offered me I objected to in my mind, ruined as it was, as unwholesome, namely, a kind of forced meat, and slices of bacon. Soon after that, I, a nervous patient, was confined in a large room with eleven or more others, nervous patients also, and servants, and certain of them occasionally raving, stamping, bawling, violent madmen. The mental agony, the distress, the actions of these wretched men, their quarrels with one another, their struggles with the servants, the servants' rude and cruel manner, my own weaknesses and follies, and the violence they brought on me, all were exposed to me, and I to them. I was confined also amongst these men, hand and foot. Often left alone for hours with two or three of them. I, weak in body, weak in mind, not able to support fear, or to control it as another, and, besides, overwhelmed by superstitious fears. This was my position for six months, until after the hay-making, and then for six months more with the difference of not being tied up. All this was under the direction of a surgeon, a physician. A surgeon attended the asylum, and surgeons came with the magistrates to inspect.[92] Now talk to me of the honesty of that class of professional men, of the respectability of physicians, of the confidence to be reposed in them! Money-making hypocrites! fawning sycophants! they deserve my curse, and they have it.

I do not recollect at any time medicine being given me; neither to purify the blood; neither as tonics; except on two occasions. No! the cheap and universal nostrum was to be

---

92 Magistrates had to inspect asylums and observe the patients several times per year to ensure that abuses were not taking place. As Perceval indicates in this account and would elaborate later, he found the inspection system to be ineffective.

ducked in the cold bath; in the depth of winter or not, no matter; no matter what my previous habits. I am thankful however even for this, that I was treated usually with more modesty here than other patients, I went usually alone, the others in a body; and generally, I had the first dip before the water had been used; but not always, and it was not always over clean.

Soon after this, boils came out on my feet and knees, and I recollect Dr. F. F. putting a black plaster over them. At that time, I imagined this was the pitch plaster to be placed over my mouth and eyes in the bath of boiling water.

At one period, I fancy about May, instead of the cold bath, I was taken to a room with a stone floor, and placed in a vapour bath. Dr. F. F. or his brother attended on two or three occasions. I thought I was to be suffocated; and when I came out safe, imagined I owed it to their prayers. My mother afterwards informed me that this treatment was undertaken at her particular request, and abandoned because they imagined it excited me. This shows how ignorant and superficial were their opinions; for indeed, I preferred it to the cold bath; it felt comfortable, the other painful. They both excited in me equal alarm. But the young doctors did not accompany me to the cold bath, and the vapour bath, no doubt, gave more trouble to the servants.

About June, if I may guess, when the buttercups and daisies were blowing in the meadows, I was taken out one or two days, walking alone with Sincerity. The second day I was fastened, in the afternoon, in a wicker chair, in the small parlour upstairs, alone. That day, one of the housekeepers, Marshall's wife, came up to me, and gave me a piece of bread, covered with jam, tasting strongly of garlick or onions. I thought she was my mother, though I did not understand

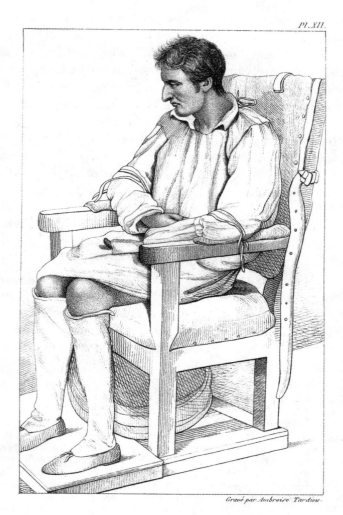

Pl. XII.

Gravé par Ambroise Tardieu.

A patient with "dementia" from Esquirol's *Des maladies mentales*, demonstrating restraints.

it, and I was desired to refuse the bread and jam as usual, but I ate it. That afternoon, or next day, I was taken to a small room adjoining, and a grey-headed gentleman I had not seen before, came in with Dr. F. and Mr. H. F. My spirits told me I was to suffer something, and gave me my option to resist it or to endure it on certain terms. I submitted; and the right temporal artery was opened until I nearly fainted.[93] I believed the gentleman was my father, and called him so. I leaned my head back on Herminet Herbert's bosom, and looking up to him, called on him by the name Jesus. After the men were gone down, he took and placed me on a close stool[94] in the room, and held me on it. I was very weak. My spirits forbade me making use of the close stool. I was then taken back and fastened in the wicker chair; then a number of delusions about singing came upon me. I imagined my temple had been closed, as the vein of a horse, by a pin and some tow; and I tried to rub the wound open, from delusion. I remained here a week or a fortnight, during which Mr. J. whom I thought my youngest brother, was occasionally allowed to come up and stay with me. He was a wild young lad, speaking in figures and hints spiritually, not understood by those around him, though I saw the spirit had a concealed meaning. I think he had a spirit of divination.

---

93   The temporal artery is the blood vessel in the head that runs in front of the ear, branching towards the forehead and across the side of the head. Although it became more controversial across the nineteenth century, bloodletting was as a treatment for many medical conditions, including madness. The Foxes professed not to put much faith in the treatment. In Perceval's second narrative, he relates that his brother told him that the operation was done to cure him of a "state of plethora," the symptoms of which included a red and full face. Perceval "saw my blood taken away in basins full." In his 1859 testimony to the Select Committee (see the introduction to this volume), Perceval would note that he "knows someone" who was permanently damaged by an operation on the temporal artery.

94   A stool over a chamber pot.

Some time after this, when my ear became swollen from extravasated blood, another slice of bread and jam tasting of garlic was given me down-stairs, after I came home from walking. Soon after, I was taken up stairs, and the same old gentleman examined my ear, and opened it with a lancet. It gave me great pain. The servants afterwards told me that great clots of blood had come out. Immediately after this, I was taken down stairs again to dinner, and treated as usual! Both times I felt very much frightened. On neither occasion had I any preparation.

I tried as soon as I was down stairs, and daily tried, to split open my ear again. What I could not do, my servant did for me. For walking out with him one forenoon, and crying out as usual, he, from his pert insolence, took upon himself to gather a switch, and to correct me with it. He struck me over the face, and the end coming round opened my wound, and the blood spirted out. He seemed alarmed and conscious, and left me on a bench in the drying ground, near which it took place, to run to the house close by for assistance, when one came, and a plaster was put on it. After that, Dr. L. who had performed both operations, examined my ear once more, but did not open it.

When I began to come round, I think the third case I exercised my judgment in, was in asking for some opening medicine.[95] Salts were given to me. A second time, my servant Hobbs forgot to ask for any, but being a make-shift kind of man, brought me two black pills he said he had got in Paris, and thought would do as well.

I have said that I asked permission not to use the cold bath from feeling conscious of its doing me injury: this was in autumn, but in the winter of 1831, when I saw through the

---

95 Laxatives.

cruelty of the system and its dupery, and called it by its right name, and struck one of the keepers. I was desired to use the cold bath again. That indignation naturally excited by a sane perception of my circumstances, by the refusal to attend to my protestations, and by my complete state of defencelessness amongst those whose characters I was impugning, was mistaken for insanity, to be treated with the infallible nostrum. So, at least, I suppose I am to take it, but *I acknowledge* I do suspect baser motives, I cannot give credit to these gentlemen for being quite so simple as they pretend to be. But this suspicion no doubt must be considered a remains of my *delusions*.

So one morning, Hobbs intimated to me that it was the doctor's desire that I should use the cold bath again; this was in January. I told my servant I had objections to it, and begged to wait till I had applied to Dr. F. F. I expected to see him during the day, but that morning he did not come. I then applied for pen, ink, and paper, to write to him, but like other requests, it was neglected: at last, on leaving my apartment to go to bed, I said to Hobbs, "will you tell Dr. F. that it is not my intention to make use of the cold bath." I had objections to it from experience, as well as from conscience; besides the disagreeableness of it at that season of the year. Next morning I was awakened early by three or four servants coming into my room. They told me they had orders to take me to the cold bath, and that I had better come quietly. I protested and argued with them. I told them I knew it was bad for me, and that it was against my conscience. What right had Dr. F. who ought, as master of an asylum, to be my protector, to force my conscience in matters indifferent to the security and peace of others? How would they reconcile it with their duty as Christians to do so? "Come, come, it is my master's orders," said Hobbs. "Yes," said I, "but you will have to answer for it before God." "Come, come, we've no time to lose." "Then," said I, "I protest against it as an Englishman, and as an English gentleman. I am placed under Dr. F., to be taken care of, not to be insulted and tyrannized over. I am not to submit, without reason, to any stupid charlatan's conceit, because I am unfortunate enough to need his control: and I call upon you to answer me before the tribunals of my own country, as well as before God, for this conduct." They then cajoled again, and advised me to come quietly—not to make resistance. I said, "don't be afraid, I will not play your master's game for him. I will not hurt any one of you, but off this bed I will not go, unless I am taken by force. When you have laid hands on me, then I will follow." They then took me by the arms and legs off the bed, and accompanied me down stairs. I called on one of them, who used to shave me occasionally, and was more good-natured than the rest, whom also I used to call Honesty, and by the name of Wynn, to be witness to the protestations, and to the force used.

I was taken down to a new bath, in every respect more cheerful and superior to that I had used the year before. It was building when I came into the mad-house. Each room was well lighted and plastered. I looked through the windows, and saw snow lying on the tiles and leads on each side. I plunged into the cold bath, and now for the first time I allowed the water to enter my mouth and drank of it. I disobeyed the voices in doing so, but it was usually a reason for me now to do any thing, if I heard a spirit forbid it. I was sorry I had never done so before, being prevented by superstitious fear, for it seemed to bring me to my senses, and to make me calm and reasonable. Since I have been at liberty I have observed that it makes the panting and agitation caused by the shock of cold water to cease: perhaps by equalizing the temperature more rapidly. After I had well bathed Hobbs opened a small door and put me under a shower-bath, the shock of which gave me the most acute pain throughout my head, as if my whole head were *one* tooth-ache. That afternoon I was placed in a private room upstairs, and I wrote to the doctor complaining of the treatment I had undergone, protesting against it, and particularly describing the pain given me by the shower-bath, the next morning I was taken down and bathed, the weather was equally severe; on the morrow I had a cold in the head and requested the servant for that cause to pass it over; he did, saying he would speak to Dr. F. Next morning in spite of my complaints, I was again bathed, and a second time placed under the shower-bath. My head was again pierced by that acute pain, and each time during the remainder of the day my head seemed on fire. I was mad now with indignation, and terrified at my danger. Fortunately soon after this I received the letter from my mother in which she states that according to my desire, she was going to remove me. Then I again stated my wish to cease from the cold bath, to Mr. H. F., (when I began to find fault with them, I was not much troubled by the visits of the other two) and he said he would speak about it, but recommended me to use the vapour bath instead; I accepted this to secure my escape from the other, as there appeared to be affectation in the offer of it, and as though it was expected from my conduct last year that I should refuse the vapour bath, when necessity would be pretended for the other.[96]

---

96   The use of the cold bath against his wishes in the winter would be one of the primary events which Perceval would later attempt to take legal action upon.

CHAPTER XX

THE DIET ALLOWED ME WAS PLAIN. In the morning and evening a basin of tea and milk poured out of a beer or water can, and four pieces of thick bread and butter. As to the manner of serving it, I was never so treated even in childhood or at school. At dinner a plain joint with potatoes and three times a week pudding, with water or small beer[97] to drink. In my opinion a few glasses of wine would have done me no harm, and I was accustomed to drink wine. Whenever I dined with the Doctor, wine was offered, but commanded by my spirits I generally refused it. I object to the manner in which my meals were given to me, more than to the nature of them. But I do not think they were quite fit for one of my habits in my situation. The patients generally used a knife and fork. I was not always allowed a knife. The servants carved the meat, and I often had great pieces of fat given me which I devoured voraciously. I remarked that after my ear had been opened I was allowed to eat as ravenously as I had previously, and no respect was paid to my diet in particular except in the middle of the year, when the three servants

97   Weak beer.

who waited on the patients in our room went away on leave of absence, and their place was supplied by three others; the old man I called my Father, another I called Honesty, and an handsome young man of a humane disposition. These three behaved very kindly, and much more respectfully. The old man when he put me to bed sometimes leant over me to kiss my forehead, saying, God bless you. Honesty used to cut me small portions of meat, and when I asked for more, shake his head considering and saying, no I think you have had enough. They were quiet and inoffensive and did not strike me except once, when the old man touched me with a stick when I was throwing myself over a style, saying, with hesitation, "I think Hobbs used to beat you for this."

But when I got my liberty I used to eat of potatoes and bread and butter most greedily. I did this in obedience to a spirit of humour, which made me try to deceive my spirits. They told me the spirits in the gentlemen round me refused their potatoes or their bread and butter for me, because I refused to obey the spirits that desired me to leave mine, and I was told if I made resolutions to use the same abstemiousness, they by doing so, would save me from much torments; it was my amusement to watch till their attention was distracted, or till I could reach the plates, and then I applied all their leavings to myself. Often of an evening I ate thus nine pieces of thick bread and butter; I never felt that I was oppressed by it. I fancy that I made myself as far as I could a perfect beast, but more particularly when my limbs were confined, and I was devouring the fat and skin put on my plate. I observed one young man, a Mr. J., often complained in a broken manner of the manner in which he was helped, and he was usually helped most unhandily; I have since suspected the fat was placed on my plate to try me, but

Chapter Twenty

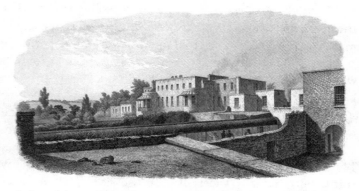

A view of the yard at Brislington as represented in the Foxes' pamphlet.

it is an even chance that the servant imagined I preferred it of a sound taste. When the table cloth was being laid for dinner, the patients were ushered into the yard where there was an alcove. Then Patience who had been standing on his legs all the forenoon, went out also into the yard; but first all the lunatics cleared the room. When I began to recover, one rainy day I refused to go into the yard preferring my seat by the fire, but after some demur I yielded, rather than cause confusion. I used to wonder also at so many madmen using their knives so harmlessly, only one day young Mr. J. cut at my legs under the table in sport with a knife. I do not think he intended to harm me, but I got up and desired to have another chair given me rather than run the risk. One evening also still later in the year, an old patient, jabbering a great deal, struck me a blow at tea, to which I replied by a smart box on the ear, which made the whole company laugh. It was seldom they did laugh. My hand struck that blow, but it was involuntary on my part, as if my hand had been moved by a violent wind. A spirit seized my arm with great rapidity, and I struck as if I was a girl. I recollect feeling grieved that the gentlemen should laugh to see a young man strike an old man. But old benevolence told me, you have done perfectly right; I was obliged to strike that old gentleman myself when he first came into the asylum, without that there is no keeping him in order.

When I say I ate my meals voraciously, I allude to the manner rather than the quantity, for I was not helped more than twice to meat and once to pudding, and once to cheese. I began eating quietly and attending to the directions of my spirits but gradually I lost all selfpossession. The day after I was bled from the temporal artery, I had a dinner of fish given me, and I was fed for many days with a wooden spoon, fastened up in my wicker chair.

CHAPTER XXI

DURING THE WHOLE PERIOD of my confinement I was never tempted to commit suicide; under my delusions I was often commanded to commit acts endangering my life and safety, but always with a view to my salvation, or that of others, and so far from any intention of self-destruction, that I expected to be raised again immediately if any evil happened to me. At Dublin I was to twist my neck, afterwards I was to suffocate myself, at Dr. F.'s I used to provoke the keepers to strike me or to throttle me. One morning after the bath, Hobbs did at my request strangle me with the strings of the straight-waistcoat after he had fastened me in the niche. He did it perhaps in sport, perhaps saying to himself, we'll see what will come of it. It did me good so far, that finding I was disappointed in the miraculous results promised to me, I desisted from requiring it. I used to throw myself over the styles, I used to throw myself forward flat on the face on the ground; and besides this the voices told me to throw myself to the right, or to the left, which I did repeatedly, and once or twice down a steep green bank round a mound in the yard to our apartment. In this I was prevented sometimes by an

old patient continually reciting incoherent sentences mingled with Latin, who mixed up his recitation with calls to
the servants indicating my danger. In all these acts I sought
a miraculous benefit. If there was any thing miraculous in
the result, it was that I escaped with whole bones. I was
not conscious of pain from the blows I received at the time,
but I knew afterwards I must have suffered pain, from the
bruises on my body. So I recollect when I sat in the niche
opposite the fireplace, I observed in the morning my feet
covered with red chilblains.[98] But my spirits said it should be
a sign to me, and that I should not feel them if I was doing
my duty to the Lord Jehovah supremely omnipotent. They
then occupied my attention by their injunctions during the
day, which I endeavoured to understand and act up to. I felt
the chilblains after breakfast, and once again after that, but
my mind was immediately occupied again, and I was rendered unconscious to the irritation.

I used repeatedly to refuse my meals in order to be
choked by their being crammed down my throat, to endure
something to the honour of the Lord Jehovah supremely
omnipotent. I was accused however of only affecting and
so to provoke choking, I tried again and again. At last one
afternoon Sincerity came to force down my meat, which I
had refused with this object. I resisted with all my power
till he literally crammed it down my gullet, bringing back
the end of the spoon with blood on it, and chipping one of
my teeth. He then came and with a coarse duster brutally
wiped my face, bringing blood from my lips or gums, and
saying, pretty boy! with a strong nasal twang. This took
place whilst all the patients were at their dinner. The Rev.
Mr. J. whom I used to call affection, got up in great agitation,

---

98   Inflammation caused by cold.

and stamped with his foot, and stretched out his trembling hands crying, "Good God, Marshall! you'll strangle him! Marshall I say!" but I made him a sign with my left hand which was fastened against the wall, meaning, be quiet, it's all for my good. I was not violent, but puerilely patient, but determined not to swallow the food but by force, and I was puzzled when my spirits told me I had done my duty so well to Sincerity that he should wipe my face so brutally afterwards.

Dr. F.'s mad-house stood in a very fine and picturesque country, and near a steep and wooded bank that bordered the river. At one elevated spot that commanded a view down the valley, a natural or artificial precipice yawned in the red soil, crowned with a small parapet, in rear of which was a small terrace and a summer house.[99] When I went out with the patients we were often conducted here. They call it the battery. The view was enchanting, but I looked down on the people working and the boats moving in the valley, with feelings that they were dead to me, and I dead to them, and yet with that painful apprehension of a dream, that I was cut off from them by a charm, by a riddle I was every minute on the point of guessing. I sat on the parapet looking down over the precipice, and Hobbs stood by me. My voices commanded me to throw myself over, that I should be immediately in heavenly places, that I was brought here to prove my faith in the Lord, that I should not be hurt if I threw myself over in his time, that if I was

---

99   A small building in an outdoor space for sitting in to enjoy good weather. The summerhouse at Brislington had three walls, with the fourth open to the elements, and a thatched roof. A later photograph of it can be seen in Clare Hickman, "The Picturesque at Brislington House, Bristol: The Role of Landscape in Relation to the Treatment of Mental Illness in the Early Nineteenth-Century Asylum," *Garden History* 33, no. 1 (2005): 47-60.

hurt I should be raised again immediately. But either the danger was too apparent, or the servant stood too near, or I had received enough rude treatment to no effect, to have less confidence in the assurances of my being a spiritual body; I did not venture. And after the second visit I did not approach the parapet, but sat in the summer house to avoid the temptation. The other patients sat on the battery. I consider it a most imprudent place to take them to.

My family chose the situation for me, partly on account of the beautiful scenery. Their kindness was ill-judged; for I have no doubt the noble views excited my spirits, awakened my imagination, and redoubled every blow of affliction, reminding me of my former health, and force of mind, and liberty. About the middle of the year, I was taken out walking with the patients, though I had not entirely given up my shouting and hallooing. We walked one after the other, I thought like a string of wild geese, nine or ten of us in a row. The hills are pretty stiff, and were, in fact, too much for me, causing my pulses to beat too rapidly. From the top of a high hill, at some distance from our abode, there was a commanding prospect to the sea, over Somersetshire into Wales: on this hill, before we descended, Samuel Hobbs cut out his initials on the soil. Now when at first I had doubted the words of my spirits, that Hobbs was my Saviour, I was desired to look on his waistcoat, and there I saw the initials S.H. marked in red silk. I was made then to understand that these initials meant Salvator Hominum;[100] and when I came to know that he was also S. Hobbs, my spirits assured me that Jesus had chosen those two names, to preserve the initials he was entitled to, and at the same time to strengthen my faith. I was directed now on the hill, and I did carve with

---

100   Latin: Savior of Man.

his stick I. upon the soil before S.H., to show my faith that he was indeed Jesus Salvator Hominum.[101]

But to resume: when I had more liberty, and was aware of my situation, I stood one day in my bed-room, before the little square glass, reflecting upon self-destruction, upon which I had always looked as a cowardly, mean, and ungenerous action; perhaps it was after having heard a patient make some painful remarks on it before the other gentlemen; perhaps it was after hearing a servant describe how one of the patients had put his head under a cart-wheel; but at the time I was considering, also, how a man could summon boldness to endure the bodily pain, as well as obliterate moral feeling; when my right arm was suddenly raised, and my hand drawn rapidly across my throat, as if by galvanism.[102] I then justified our law, which acquits an insane man from the verdict of *felo de se*;[103] and I determined not to advert to the subject again, seeing that I had not control over my spirits, until I was free from provocation: in which resolution I persevered.

---

101   In Latin, Jesus begins with an I.

102   Electricity. Luigi Galvani was an Italian scientist who studied the effects of electricity on the body after causing the limbs of a dead frog to twitch. Galvani's experiments influenced Mary Shelley's *Frankenstein*.

103   The term for one found guilty of ending their own life.

CHAPTER XXII

NOW WITH REGARD TO MY TREATMENT, I have to make at first two general observations, which apply, I am afraid, too extensively to every system of management yet employed towards persons in my condition. First, the suspicion and the fact of my being incapable of reasoning correctly, or deranged in understanding, justified apparently every person who came near me, in dealing with me also in a manner contrary to reason and contrary to nature. These are strong words; but in the minutest instances I can, alas! prove them true. Secondly, my being likely to attack the rights of others gave these individuals license, in every respect, to trample upon mine. My being incapable of feeling, and of defending myself, was construed into a reason for giving full play to this license. Instead of my understanding being addressed and enlightened, and of my path being made as clear and plain as possible, in consideration of my confusion, I was committed, in really difficult and mysterious circumstances, calculated of themselves to confound my mind, even if in a sane state, to unknown and untried hands; and I was placed amongst strangers, without introduction, explanation, or exhortation. Instead of great scrupulousness being observed in depriving me of any liberty or privilege, and of the exercise of so much choice and judgment as might be conceded to me with safety;—on the just ground, that for the safety of society my most valuable rights were already taken away, on every occasion, in every dispute, in every argument, the assumed premise immediately acted upon was, that I was to yield, my desires were to be set aside, my few remaining privileges to be infringed upon, for the convenience of others. Yet I was in a state of mind not likely to acknowledge even the justice of my confinement, and in a state of defencelessness calculated to make me suspicious, and jealous of any further invasion of my natural and social rights: but this was a matter that never entered into their consideration.

Against this system of downright oppression, enforced with sycophantish adulation and affected pity by the doctor, adopted blindly by the credulity of relations, and submitted to by the patients with meek stupidity, or vainly resisted by natural but hopeless violence, I had to fight my way for two years, wringing from my friends a gradual but tardy assent to the most urgent expostulations: not from the physicians; their law is the same for all qualities and dispositions, and their maxim to clutch and hold fast.

The first step adopted towards me by my friend, Captain ———, in Dublin, was injudicious and indelicate. If I had been incoherent, I had hitherto only rendered myself ridiculous; and if, by one act, I had run the risk of injuring my person, it was also evident that I had relinquished my purpose at the request of his family. I trace my ruin to the particular trials, to the surprise, the confusion, the puzzle, which the sudden intrusion of a keeper brought upon me. But at that time, unfortunately, I did not consider my dignity so much as my relationship to the Almighty, as his redeemed servant, bound in gratitude, and from self-abasement, to exercise forbearance and humility. If it be replied, My ruin might have been brought about another way; I answer, I do not know what might have been, but I know what did take place.

The first symptoms of my derangement were, that I gazed silently on the medical men who came to me, and resolutely persisted in acts apparently dangerous. No doubt there were also symptoms of bodily fever. But from that moment to the end of my confinement, men acted as though my body, soul, and spirit were fairly given up to their control, to work their mischief and folly upon. My silence, I suppose, gave consent. I mean, that I was never told, such and such things we are going to do; we think it advisable to administer such and such medicine, in this or that manner; I was never asked. Do you want any thing? do you wish for, prefer any thing? have you any objection to this or to that? I was fastened down in bed; a meagre diet was ordered for me; this and medicine forced down my throat, or in the contrary direction; my will, my wishes, my repugnances, my habits, my delicacy, my inclinations, my necessities, were not once consulted, I may say, thought of. I did not find the respect paid usually even to a child. Yet my mind was at first sound, except as far as it was deceived by preternatural injunctions; in a certain respect, it remained sound throughout my illness, so that it faithfully recorded the objects and the events that took place around me; but I looked to the inspirations I received for the interpretation of them. If at any time my ear could have been closed to my delusions, I was then fit to be at liberty; but the credit I gave to my delusions, rather than to my judgment, was my disease. I was not, however, once addressed by argument, expostulation, or persuasion. The persons round me consulted, directed, chose, ordered, and force was the unica and ultima ratio[104] applied to me. If I were insane, in my resolution to be silent, because I was sure that neither of the doctors, or of my friends, would understand my motives, or give credit to facts they had not themselves experienced; they were surely no less insane, who, because of my silence, forgot the use of their own tongues,—who, because of my neglect of the duties I owed to them, expunged from their consciences all deference to me; giving up so speedily and entirely all attempt at explanation; all hope of sifting the cause of my delusions; all hope of addressing my reason with success; all hope of winning me to speak. If I needed medicine and light diet, still, I say to myself, surely that was not all; surely air and exercise, and water, and occupation or amusement, and a little solid food, would have done me no harm. Certainly, if they wanted to ensure a case for medicine, and broths, and ultimately for a lunatic asylum, the neglect of my nature, as an animal and intellectual being, was consistent. These two poor gentlemen in Dublin were, however, comparatively innocent. *They went like a donkey blindfolded*, round and round in the mill, the same to them whether the cord that draws up the water was broken or not.[105] They, with whom I had to do in England, were perverse as well as infatuated. There, when I began to understand my wants, to know my rights, to claim them, to upbraid, remonstrate, threaten, in order to procure respect for them, the reply was still the same. "The doctors advise, and your family are

104 Latin: unique and final reason.

105 Some mills were powered not by water or wind but by a horse or donkey walking in circles around a central post.

bound to follow blindly their advice; and you must submit, whether or no."

My position was in every respect more depressing when I came to Dr. F—'s. I was no longer in rooms that I had chosen, but in a new place, to which I had been removed without my will having been consulted, and left there without explanation. This gave inlet to, and confirmed the delusion, that I was no longer a free agent, but under the control of beings superiorly enlightened. I may say, that I met with no persuasion, explanation, or exhortation throughout the time of my residence here; but, to speak more strictly, no remonstrance was addressed to me in a manner befitting my age, character, or situation. I have already mentioned how I was disappointed in my brother's conduct; he made light of my delusions, and I said to myself, he must be a perfect fool, to know what power of mind I had, and to think I am acting without a very strong cause. After being treated with so little reflection by him, I was not surprised at strangers behaving in the same manner; but, in truth, whilst they were pitying my folly, I was shocked at, and pitying theirs. My delusions had rendered me imbecile, but I was not aware of it; and they addressed me as a child, and I did not understand them, because I knew I was a man.

Dr. F—'s system was to class all the errors of his patients under the head of imagination. A safe and plausible term, used to catch others, and to disguise their own ignorance; at the same time, that it augured little of respect or hope to the patient, the effects of whose imagination on him were often as real, as the impression of sensible objects on the supercilious doctor. It was not likely, therefore, that I should confide the difficulties of my mind to men who, by slighting the origin of them, betrayed their presumption, whilst affecting excellent acuteness.

The doctor's manner of address to me, and that of others, always puzzled me, and made it difficult for me to act or to reply: it was coupled, too, with a kind of half-and-half manner, as if my sincerity were mistrusted, which corroborated the communications my spirits made to me, that they came to try me; and when I regained better health, became very offensive. Sometimes, if I called out aloud, the young doctor would assume a winning smile, and put his finger playfully to his mouth: once he asked, "What do you mean by saying you are the redeemed of the Lord Jehovah, supremely omnipotent? don't you think that I am? I hope I am, and these gentlemen too." The tone and manner rendered these questions perplexing, and would have excited my ridicule, if my mind had not been too much occupied to give way to it. The reply perhaps most on my tongue was, Do you take me for a child? do you think I do and suffer all I have gone through without reason? They suited their behaviour to that which I appeared to be, taking advantage of my weakness, instead of correcting it. Because I did not respect myself, they disrespected me; whereas they should have brought me to my senses by greater reserve and respect. They forgot that, amidst all my lunatic childishness and simplicity, I was a grown-up man, and probably knew not myself. And if it is true of any creature, that he knoweth not of what spirit he is, it is strikingly true of a lunatic.

The first and most blameable error of the doctor was to place me in a noisy and crowded parlour, the common sitting-room of the madmen. He a physician; I, a nervous patient, and a gentleman. The conduct of my relations was as blameable, to leave me so far from home, under the guidance of men, complete strangers to me and to them, and my inferiors in rank and profession, careless or wittingly exposing me to so much rude contact and observation.[106] Had I been lunatic on any ordinary subject, it would have been their duty to have reflected, that in all probability my conscience was affected, and that I might require a friend and a clergyman, to whom to confide my troubles. But they knew that my mind was deranged by over study on religion. And they left me exposed to strangers, and what is still more humbling to human nature, and to the pride and religion of my country, they who stand in no mean situation for wealth, talents, rank, or morality—they who are not merely fashionable professors of religion, and many of whom are even zealous in evangelical opinions,—took so little thought, as to consign my soul and spirit, in the hour of my utmost need, to the absolute control of a physician who was a sectarian,[107] whilst my body was committed to his menials. Dr. F. had been a member of the Society of Friends; and, naturally enough, the spirit of the burlesque doctrines of that sect crept into his system, where they only warred with the interests of the patient; so that when, in the next year, I complained of the degrading footing of familiarity on which I had been placed with the domestics, and of the conduct in which they had been allowed towards me, he replied to me, in a letter to this effect, "Had not Jesus made us all equal?"[108]

---

106 While Dr. Fox's asylum was segregated by class, the employees themselves, including the physician, would have been from a lower class than Perceval.

107 One dedicated to a schismatic religious group.

108 The Society of Friends—also known as the Quakers—played an outsized role in the development of the asylum in the United Kingdom. William Tuke popularized the moral treatment that dominated asylums through the

Placed amongst strangers, the idea of opening my thoughts and unburdening my spirit to them scarcely entered my mind. Confession and confidence were acts from which, however salutary, I was precluded. Deranged and imbecile as I was, I was not yet so brutal as those who left me, and exposed me to the temptation of unveiling the secrets of my conscience; of betraying the dealings of God with me to individuals unknown to me; of laying myself open to their secret and prying curiosity; and my weaknesses, first, to their inward ridicule, then to their outward mocking;—to be forced to run this hazard, or to have my mind preyed upon by its agonies, was cruel. At that time I shrunk even from crying out the sentences the spirits dictated to me, acknowledging my ruin. Since then, my sufferings, my despair of being attended to, have hardened me, and made me reckless.

When I began first to write to my mother and my brother, complaining of my situation, and aware of my state, my feelings were acute in this respect, and my instances earnest and repeated that my correspondence should be private. Delicacy towards my family, if only that, dictated this. I received no attention.[109] The same bigotted credulity that abandoned my person and soul to the doctor's management, abandoned also the secrets of my heart to his impertinent examination. I cannot describe the hatred with which the

---

mid-century, and Tuke's York Retreat would have been a model for Brislington House. Ostensibly, the system involved treating patients with kindness and providing wholesome structure. While this was clearly an improvement on earlier, more brutal treatments, Perceval's narrative makes plain that the system retained both physical punishment and, more troubling for him, a tone of condescension.

109 Later in life, Perceval would campaign for the privacy of patient's mail—except in cases where a lady was likely to write scandalous things.

recollection of this conduct still inspires me: then I hated, I despised, I was enraged, I became hardened. I loathed myself for keeping any terms with my relations and those around me. In the end, I scoffed at religion; I blasphemed the name and nature of God. The doctor alone benefited; for his benefit it was designed. Liable to his subtle misrepresentation, I concealed and disguised my feelings, or wrote for his inspection, braving his malice and duplicity. My real distresses I left to time or chance to take away, or to unravel. I was brutalized.

Thus, in a state of derangement, I was abandoned to my fate, and so condemned, that I could not seek health by sane conduct. I could not recover sanity, but by ways which can alone be justified by insanity; from which I shrunk, even insane: ways, which the very nature of a sound understanding, the very nature of humane feeling, make impossible. But this is one example only. When I grew older in my afflictions, I found that no patient could escape from his confinement in a truly sound state of mind, without lying against his conscience, or admitting the doctrine, that deception and duplicity are consistent with a sound conscience. Those who do otherwise are not sane, they are living in a lie. But what does that signify? they are good subjects, and the doctor's best friends.

CHAPTER XXIII

I RECOLLECT, when I first began to be aware of the insults and affronts put upon me with my daily food, and felt the impropriety of my situation, I still did not accuse or lay the charge to the doctor indiscriminately; but I determined to seek information before I judged. Mankind will, I think, consider it an affecting sight, when they behold a young gentleman, at the dawn of returning light, awakened to the consciousness of the cruelties around him; of the advantage that had been taken of his darkness; of the degrading treatment he was exposed to, yet examining and hesitating before he condemned. I reasoned with myself, for I was without a friend,—first as a citizen, then as a private individual: as an Englishman, I laid charge to the government, to the magistrates; more especially to the prelates, who supinely abandoned the trust committed to them, over the souls of the diseased members of the church, to the doctors, who serve as eyes to the magistrates.[110] But

---

110 Perceval would later campaign for increased involvement of religious officials, or prelates, in asylum monitoring and care—a controversial opinion

these were evils I could not remedy. As a private individual, I knew not which most to blame, the doctor or my family. I recollected the two or three first days of treatment; my private parlour, my meals neatly served, the silver forks, &c., and I doubted whether, for my misconduct, I had not been degraded; and had my family been made acquainted with the change, or was the doctor imposing upon them. Therefore, in great distress of mind and anxiety, I wrote to my mother, stating my complaints, asking if they aware of my position, and insisting upon a private apartment, and a servant to attend on me alone. Part of the answer I received was to the effect, that my elder brother *thought* that I was to have a room to myself, or that I was to be allowed to go to my bed-room. I was shocked at the indifference which this uncertainty betrayed. When I wrote that letter, I still considered more the evil effect my misfortunes might have had on the inclinations of my mother and sisters to believe the doctrines of the Row heresy, to which I yet adhered, than my own necessities. I put several questions connected with my peace of mind. I received no answer to them. What I wrote, I saw on the paper, or heard dictated before I put it down; often printing it in capital or other letters, as I saw it printed. But I wrote in trouble and agony,—abruptly and without much connexion; which was not surprising, for I was not alone.*[III]

within the Alleged Lunatics' Friend Society. He also argued that the current system of monitoring was flawed, and failed to hold abusive doctors accountable.

III   [Perceval's note] *The above was written in Paris last year from memory. Since my return to London, I find, on referring to papers I have preserved, that my first letter was written on or about the 29th of November; for I have a copy of a letter I commenced on that day, which I afterwards altered: it was to my elder brother. This letter was detained until about the 22nd of December; for I find the copy of an envelope, dated the 19th of December, and directed to my brother, in which I complain of the detention*

Chapter Twenty-Three

I was then in the small parlour with three other gentlemen with whom for a few days past I had been allowed to dine and pass the evening there; probably selected on account of our better behaviour, and because the room below was too crowded. I wrote the letter under the promise three times given me before I sent it, by Dr. F. F., that it should not be opened. I knew that I was expressing myself without control over my feelings, and my delicacy and modesty shrunk from what I wrote being disclosed to strangers, or pried into by self-interested, empirical, or idle curiosity. I had also other reasons that I did not like Dr. F. to be aware that I was suspecting him of dishonesty, or to charge him with it without grounds, and I might betray family matters. My letter however was opened by old Dr. F.; this was communicated to me the day after I had delivered it into the hands of Dr. F. F., when dining with the latter and his wife. My first expression after that of astonishment was, "Well, I am glad of it," for I only felt, then the Dr. knows

---

of that letter, and enclose one to my mother, written about the 11th of December. These letters, and others, I have thrown into an appendix to this volume, not to break the thread of the text, and to prevent any further delay in this publication.

I acknowledge I am confounded at the bare-faced impudence of the doctor in detaining my first letter so long. I do not know whether to attribute it to cowardice, — from a consciousness that I was not entirely wrong in my accusations, and to his knowledge of the security and impunity with which he could treat me so unjustly, — or to his habitual indifference to complaints of the patients against his system, from the infatuated prepossession that his asylum was a second paradise. The excuse that he made to me was, that he hoped I should see fit to change my sentiments before I wrote to my mother, that he was loath to send a letter that might wound their feelings.

I know what I know. But in this world I must talk of a supreme and benevolent Providence, and of certain individuals being honourable and sincere, or be ejected from society. I know too little, or too much; too much, without more courage to act according to my understanding; too little, without more understanding to put my knowledge in practice.

[Editor's note] Perceval does not attach these letters in an appendix to this first, anonymous edition of his memoirs. His second edition, however, contains much correspondence.

the state of my feelings not by my fault. But I afterwards felt exposed, insulted, indignant, betrayed, when I recollected other parts of the letter, and foresaw that I could have no peace in communicating with my family, unless I was secure of the privacy of my correspondence. If they had not been deceived, they were perhaps unworthy of my concern. I insisted on that privacy as much for their sakes as mine: but although repeatedly mentioned by me, my request was not even once alluded to; yet even although it might have been an excessively extravagant request, if it gave me peace of mind, it was right to have attended to it. This silent, and as I felt it, contumelious contempt of my most earnest request, and expostulations, repeated on several occasions nearly drove me mad. If the show of an argument for not acceding to so simple and usual a wish had been given me, that would have proved attention at least, and some sort of respect: but to be passed over in silence, and apparently for the very reason, that a reason ought to have been given, because I was myself bereft of reason. I could not make it out, and I could not endure it. Now after these things, when I upbraided my family for their contempt, they argued from my accusation that I was a madman; because how could I imagine that such kind, excellent, affectionate relatives, wished to show me contempt. Not reflecting—and I wrote back to them—that contempt is contempt, but that the wish to show contempt is flattering to the pride and vanity of the object of it, because he knows that the contempt is affected. Henceforward, however, this was the hopeful tribunal to which I had to appeal for three years, they judging themselves and their conduct by their own excellent opinion of themselves, and me as a madman, for accusing such excellence, and refusing me my appeal to a jury, my appeal to law, my rights and privileges, on the plea that I should at length confess my errors, and be sorry to have so dealt with such excellent people, who left me in the mean time to pine and rot in a lunatic asylum.[112]

To return to my letter, I obtained also, three times, a promise from Dr. F. F. that it should be forwarded immediately. Consider my wretched circumstances, consider my state of mind, my state of health, the resentment I felt at the treatment I had already endured, the acute suffering that treatment still occasioned me, my suspense, believing my letter to be sent, and no answer; and then you may conceive my danger, my exasperation, my despair, when on inquiry, many weeks after the letter was written, I found it had not been sent. Dr. F., with empirical sagacity, wanted me to write something more connected, to alter the expressions concerning his asylum more favourably. Yet on his son's deprecating my sending such a letter to my family, whilst I was yet writing it, and when I asked him for his last promise to send it without reading it, I showed him the words which I had written, explaining the reason why I preferred sending my scrawl as it was, to correcting it; whilst I covered with my hands the rest of the letter. My reasons were, that my brother's considering my hand-writing and my style, might try to find out for me the cause of, or the mystery of my malady. Poor fool! I might as well have written to the stones, or to the winds. They showed me no real desire to inquire, no delicacy, no beauty of feeling.

They who have not been confined in a lunatic asylum, cannot conceive the dreadful and cruel suspense that delay,

---

112 Again, this would form the basis of much of Perceval's later advocacy: the inability of the accused or recovered lunatic to appeal their diagnosis and incarceration.

and not only the neglect, but the refusal of every day civilities, together with inattention to just and obvious complaints, occasion. They do not know our wants and fears, because they do not know the danger we are in. They may judge our danger, however, from what these men do; and from what they have done, they may judge what they dare to do: being encompassed, even more than a king, with a hollow impunity, and clothed in the deepest hypocrisy. They who have not endured this confinement do not know how the very suspicion of being a lunatic, coupled with being cut off from all pecuniary resources, shuts the minds of others against sympathy, impedes the proffer of assistance and the exercise of protection, and aught but the show of pity. Neither how it embarrasses the suppliant in his applications for redress, awakens anxiety, excites mistrust, and closes the door of his hopes; whilst he finds himself left defenceless to the sarcasm and persecutions of those he is accusing. This is an awful peril for a man in a sound mind to be exposed to, lest he become deranged; lest he be tempted to violence, *the object* of his tormentors, which would then be construed into an open act of insanity; and if not immediately accepted as damning proof, by imbecile magistrates, at least cruelly try the mind, by tantalizing the expectations. How much more fearful is such a trial for one who knows that he cannot plead innocence of lunacy; one who, in mind and bodily health, is weak, and thereby more exposed than another to follow a wrong course; exposed to suffer even from treatment which men in sound health might almost laugh at, still more from that which he dreads from having experienced it, and against which he is exasperated; and also, still more liable than the other to lose that gift, lately lost, so dear now, being newly restored to him,—the gift of a sound mind, and convalescent health; perishing again from want of wholesome communion, shattered by assault, or insidiously undermined.

By this time I had broken off all friendly intercourse with the Drs. F. He had explained to me that he acted with the sanction of my family, and they, by his guidance: and my eldest brother in a letter stated, only (so loosely had he acted) that he thought some agreement had been made with regard to my having a private apartment; but on further reflection, as my mind grew stronger, considering my rights and my state more accurately, I concluded that the doctor was responsible to me, that he had forfeited claim to my respect, and deserved great blame, both as a physician and as a man of honour and gentlemanly feeling, in exposing me in a state of nervous excitement and great weakness, to the violence, confusion, and open observation of the society and servants in his common room: particularly when he knew my name, and the kind of society in which I had lived, to which I had been brought up; and the circumstances of my illness. As my fall was great, so was my trial severe, and his conduct the more highly to be censured. But the year before, an officer in the army, now to be put under the sticks, the fists, the knees of his menials, at their discretion: deranged through enthusiastically religious principles, and left amongst a motley group of blaspheming, infidel, and irreligious lunatics. Yesterday a gentleman, moving in the most refined and honourable circles, to-day in a room full of fanatics coarse even by habits, and of vulgar education; to select such a time to heap all these painful trials and cruel contrasts upon me! But no matter; the ruin of the soul has been accomplished; the work of villany has been done; what is now the use of complaint, what the use of remonstrating

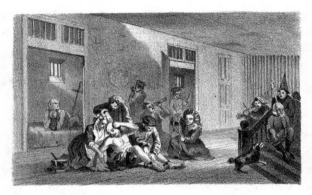

Haskell's asylum exposé included a rendition of the final plate
from William Hogarth's famous Rake's Progress, which depicts
a rich young heir's path through debauchery to Bedlam.

against such bare-faced and impudent mockery: moreover, I
did not feel it then; I could not resent their cruelties; I was
overwhelmed by other afflictions: the waves that wash over
the body of a drowned man shock and lift the limbs, it is
true; but they fall again on the sands, listless and impassible.
Be it supposed, I did not feel it then.

The want of feeling with which we were treated, however,
is difficult to be credited, and the degree of folly to which it
proceeded, scarcely to be imagined. Communications, when
they came from our families, were made to us in the presence
of the rest, vivâ voce.[113] Letters were given to us to read, and
materials to write, in public. I received no tidings from my
family, as near as I can guess, for three months: I understood
afterwards, from my mother, when released, that in this, as
in other parts of her conduct, equally contrary to nature and
reason, she obeyed the advice of the doctor. They had got a
stranger into their nets, and they were determined to keep

---

113   Out loud.

him all to themselves. I am surprised at their self-sufficiency and impertinence. The natural result of this neglect was to produce in my mind surprise, wonder, a sense of strangeness in my situation, and alarm, to find a satisfactory clue to which, I had nothing but a disordered imagination to draw upon, which supplied me, as I have indicated, with ludicrous and horrible ideas enow.[114] I was led also to entertain a mean opinion of myself, and to condemn myself by too severe a judgment. So that when I began to address my friends, I was at a loss to know how to approach them. What was I to augur from their silence; had they cast me off? did they look on me as a reprobate? did they scout me?[115]

At last, a message in a letter, or a letter to me, was delivered to me in the common room one forenoon. It was from my mother. Either on that, or on a subsequent occasion later in the year, I was asked if I would write an answer. I applied to my spirits, as usual, for guidance as to the feelings I was to express, the acts I was to perform. I hallooed aloud, and behaved boisterously by their direction. I got pen, ink, and paper brought to me, and a table; kicked them over; had them replaced; and at length wrote to my mother to this effect: "that I was so happy where I was: that I loved the people so about me; that I longed to come to E——, and to bring Herminet Herbert with me," and I alluded to my spiritual friend, Mr. Waldony. I wrote with great perplexity, and opposition from many of the spirits. Unfortunately, my family were too willing to believe this silly rhapsody, although there were a few words that might have afforded them a clue to the truth; and I was informed, when released, that the contents of that letter greatly influenced them in

---

114 Enough.

115 To scout is to mock or scorn.

rejecting the complaints I made, when I began really to appreciate my situation. I did not call to mind what I had written, until they recalled it to my recollection; and I was then very angry that my family had never frankly alluded to my previous statements, in order that I might have come to an explanation. I wrote two or three short letters in the same style: in the last, I begged my mother to excuse me from replying to her, as it gave me great pain. I then did not hear from her for a long time, and I was afraid she understood that receiving the letters she wrote gave me pain. My meaning was, that I could not answer her for the contest of my spirits; for many came to write for me, or to dictate to me, and I became agitated, and vexed which to put faith in, which to choose. In other words, I imagine it was a contest of mind, between the spirit of a right understanding and the spirits of delusion. Had I been alone, I might by chance have written soundly, my senses being calmer and more collected. But besides the delusions and the simplicity which obscured my intellect, I doubt not that my sorrows and sufferings, called for actions and expressions I unconsciously shrunk from before strangers; and if I behaved in an unusual manner, if my agitation made me leave the table, or lay down my pen; if I wandered in my attention, one of the servants would come and incite me to go on, or take away pen, ink, and paper together, saying, "what's the use of giving it to you if you make no use of it;" or "come, come I think you have written enough for to-day;" then another entering the room, and staring at me, cried out, "has he finished the letter yet," and if not, then "take it away, take it away from him; he'll be all the day about it."

CHAPTER XXIV

IN JUNE, about the time of hay-making, my eldest brother, on his way from T—— after his election, called to see me.[116] I was unfastened, led into another patient's room, and dressed in a new suit of clothes, like a boy at a private school, and taken into the entrance room to see him. After speaking to him, some gooseberry pie was offered to me; and then I walked out with my brother and the keeper; tried to throw myself over the stiles as usual, and came home. Next day, I again walked out with him; he took me to a seat, where he asked me to explain him a proposition in Euclid, which I comprehended perfectly, but was prevented by my spirits from following consecutively; it seemed to me as if I had other business; and I thought he was come to try me, and was inspired to know all my thoughts. From the seat I drew a sketch, with some difficulty, partly guided by the spirits, partly of my own handy-work; and I desired him to give it to my elder sister. My brother took leave of me in the evening, in the common room, at tea time. I was then fastened up in

---

116 His brother Spencer served several terms as a Member of Parliament. While John was incarcerated, Spencer was elected in Tiverton.

the niche. I was told by the voices that he would have taken me to E———, which my heart was set upon, if I had performed one extravagant act or another, which I had failed in, or refused to do.

Before my brother's arrival, or soon after, my mother had desired the doctor to supply me with books, and had written to know what books I should like to have sent to me. She had also desired them to propose to me to draw and to learn the flute; Mr. H. F. asked me to read Virgil with him, and Dr. F. F. suggested the occupation of turning.[117] I sent for a Euclid and my Hebrew bible; I agreed to try my hand at drawing, and a school-boy's copy-book and one pencil were given to me. Was it intended to turn me to ridicule? to provoke me to exercise my judgment? or, was it from simplicity and hypocrisy; pretending to do what they cared nothing about? As to the music-master, I did not believe that the offer was sincere. I thought that they came to try me, and at any rate that it was of no use, for though I could understand what I read, and might blow on the flute, I knew I could not apply to study, until I understood the calls of the spirits, and how to follow or reconcile their directions. In the same season, I was astonished at Dr. F. F. proposing to me the use of a turning machine:[118] and I could not believe his sincerity, for I knew the first day I should put my finger where it would be crushed, in obedience to a voice of one kind or of another. I asked for Gibbon's Roman History, but it was never brought to me, and as they fought off from this request, my suspicions were increased. Long after, when books were again offered to me, I again asked for the History of the Decline and Fall of the Roman

---

117   Crafting with a lathe.

118   Lathe.

Empire, instead of which I was presented to my amusement
with the history of the Lew-chew Islands.[119] But, Herminet
Herbert (Hobbs) exercised a summary control over all these
petty occupations, and on one pretence or another often
took my pencil and books away from me, or prevented me
bringing them down-stairs. Small as these means were, they
doubtless aided my recovery; occupying me on realities,
and for a time rescuing me from sloth, apathy, and idleness.
It was one of my first complaints by letter, that they were
taken away; and, I think, the only one that was immediately
attended to. These attentions, such as they were, I owed
chiefly to my mother's persevering instances, together with
other particular alterations. Unfortunately, I did not know
until I was released, how much I had been even thus far
indebted to her.

My brother was evidently agonised at my appearance.
His visit gave me self-confidence, and insured me some
respect. More advantage might have resulted from it,
had my situation been more becoming. But a visit of this
kind, and the style of delivery in which communications
were made from our families, and the patients requested
to reply to them, are instances of the mockery and treachery of such a system in a mad-house. By placing you in
an unnatural and cruel situation, and at the same time
counselling your friends to keep aloof from you, in presence and in letter, they create the feelings which render
it impossible for a man in a sound mind to receive intelligence from them at last, without extreme agitation: then
they abruptly communicate that intelligence, or hand the
letter to the patient, and neither consulting his modesty

---

119   A nineteenth-century English name for the Ryukyu Islands, a chain of
what are now Japanese Islands.

or his distress, deny him a little retirement to read these lines in private. His feelings, at a time that he is declared incapable of controlling them, are thus called upon, in the very circumstances, from the cruelty of which he ought to have been preserved, by those from whom he hears, for which they ought at least to express their sympathy, and regret, if not atone and apologize. But no, the letter contains a mere meagre account of every day occurrences; cold, unmeaning, paltry trivialities, trifling with the time and tone of a mind whose imagination is strung up to the highest pitch of delicate and romantic enthusiasm. The violence, or agitation, or ridiculous conduct that ensues, is then attributed to the receipt of the letter, instead of to the brutal heedlessness with which it is delivered. But this is in favour of the doctor. Another apparent cause is given for withholding at least, if not denying altogether, one rational mean of a patient's recovery; and however specious may be their conduct, and their excuses to mankind and to themselves, their end is to make money, not to make whole; and their system is adapted in one way or another to this end: whilst the essential interests, the mental wants of the inmates of their prisons are neglected. It stands to reason. Tie an active limbed, active minded, actively imagining young man in bed, hand and foot, for a fortnight, drench him with medicines, slops, clysters;[120] when reduced to the extreme of nervous debility, and his derangement is successfully confirmed, manacle him down for twenty-four hours in the cabin of a ship; then for a whole year shut him up from six, A.M. to eight, P.M. regardless of his former habits, in a room full of strangers, ranting, noisy,

---

120 Clysters are rectally administered medicines; "slops" likely refers the unappetizing liquified diet spoon-fed to someone ill.

quarrelsome, revolting, madmen; give him no tonic med-icines,[121] no peculiar treatment or attention, leave him to a nondescript domestic, now brushing his clothes, sweep-ing the floors, serving at table, now his companion out of doors, now his bed-room companion; now throwing him on the floor, kneeling on him, striking him under all these distressing and perplexing circumstances; debar him from all conversation with his superiors, all communication with his friends, all insight into their motives, every impression of sane and well-behaved society! surprise him on all occa-sions, never leave harassing him night or day, or at meals; whether you bleed him to death, or cut his hair, show the same utter contempt for his will or inclination; do all in your power to crush every germ of self-respect that may yet remain, or rise up in his bosom; manacle him as you would a felon; expose him to ridicule, and give him no opportunity of retirement or self-reflection; and what are you to expect. And whose agents are you; those of God or of Satan? And what good can you reasonably dare to expect? and whose profit is really intended?

Gentlemen of England, the system I have described is not only the system of English men, it is the disgrace of English surgeons, of English physicians. It is practised or connived at by the innocent simplicity of that race of presuming upstarts, who in various guises admitted by your condescension to terms of familiarity, sit at your tables, hiding their conceit in a false humility and in silky smiles; whilst they ape your manners and dupe your generosity. Be assured, whoever ye are, who have to deal with children or lunatics, if you are not looking after them yourselves, you are not respecting them. The doctors know that, and take

---

121 Medicines designed to strengthen and sustain healthy function.

advantage of it, to construe your disrespect into worse even than it is. Their servants take advantage of it. Bystanders draw false conclusions from it, much rather the poor object of it. His nature resents it; though he is not always aware of anything but his delusions: and his delusions contending with his feelings for the mastery over him, make him a madman. His self-respect, also, for so he respected himself partly for your sakes, is destroyed; and he delivers himself up to every grovelling thought and lewd idea, reckless on account of *your* ingratitude; even if his weakness and total want of wholesome exercise, wholesome occupation, and wholesome repose, does not render such a surrender inevitable. If, however, he has sense to resent consciously your desertion, he has also ten to one the high-mindedness to do it by scorn, contempt, and silence on his part; perhaps he does so by expressions of hatred and attempts at violence in your presence, devoid of discretion, and impotent over his revenge. These the doctor, consciously or not, easily gets you to interpret into signs of the complaint, when they are in truth the signs of his devilish treatment, and of the patient's unguarded honesty: which, also, a few respectful words of repentance from you might make vanish like the morning mists. Not however, if you repent only to offend again; if you mock at one who, whatever may be the source, is preternaturally enlightened. I am sure that no lunatic who has undergone the trials I describe, can meet his family on terms of cordiality, but through practising dissimulation, or through being a simpleton. At this distance of time, I cannot forgive my family the guilt they incurred by their abandonment of me. I am at a loss to find any argument which will justify me in doing so: I dare not expect to be able to do so. But if haply perfection requires this moral excellence, by what happy fortune are you entitled to look for it in the inmates of a lunatic asylum?

I have complained that the behaviour adopted towards me, was calculated to humour the state of mind I was then in, not to correct. The servant, for instance, whom I used to call Jesus, and Herminet Herbert, ran with me, jumped, joked, walked arm in arm with me, rattled the spoons in my face as he put them into the cupboard, pulled me by the nose, &c. &c. If I was not insensible to the impropriety of this familiarity, at least, I could not express my sense of it. But it will be evident, this was not the way to correct a gentleman's diseased mind. This conduct may be partly accounted for by having been placed under a quondam Quaker,[122] to whom in theory and in practice, as far as it only interfered with others, and suited his interests, perfect equality of rich and poor was a matter of faith. There was, however, this unfairness in it, that I observed the joke ceased whenever the domestic had had enough of it. The lunatic's presence of mind and tranquillity might be broken in upon, but not so the keeper's. There was but one step from joking with them to violence and objurgation.[123] Later in the year, a young handsome lad used to invite me to box with him every evening in my bed-room, striking me in sport a few blows: at length, I expressed a kind of awkward resentment at it. I have perhaps written enough on this subject.

---

122   That is, one who had once been a Quaker, possibly with the implication that he had been tossed out.

123   Scolding.

CHAPTER XXV

ONE SUNDAY MORNING, old Dr. F. entered the common room as usual; and on his entrance I, who was tied hand and foot, sang the psalm, "O be joyful," &c. to the edification of those present. The doctor tottered up to me on his cane, and argued against the impropriety of my conduct in singing, in such a place, such a psalm on a Sunday morning. This was the kindest and most reasonable address made to me during my imbecility in that madhouse. But it was lost upon me, because I did not believe it sincere. My spirits had told me to sing the psalm in his honor, and purposely to please him. That I was not to mind what he said, because he spoke so to see if I preferred serving God or him; and that he was really delighted to hear me sing it, as a proof that I was returning to a sense of my duty to the Lord Jehovah; and trying to fulfil my mission as an angel who was to sing his praises. Sunday morning appeared to me an additional reason. His using that argument aided the spirits in deluding me. Therefore as soon as he re-entered the room from the yard, I pealed forth again, "O be joyful in the Lord, all ye lands," though not so decidedly. His word helped to make me doubt the word of the spirits.

One forenoon, after I was allowed to walk out in the common room and yard, Mr. F. F. whilst standing near me and three other patients, asked me suddenly before them, "Pray, Mr.—was it your father who was shot in the house of Commons?"[124] I do not know whether I replied; but I recollect being greatly troubled by my spirits to make a reply, though inwardly at peace. I then looked silently in the faces of the bystanders, and then turned my back on him, and walked away to meditate on what had occurred, alone. I will not say what I feel now. The next part of the treatment I will allude to, is my having been walked about the grounds and the country in a state of insanity. The chief thing to be desired in the treatment of an insane person (as any but charlatans would have inferred from the name they give them, *"nervous patient"*[125]) is quiet, peace, security; security from intrusion, observation, exposure. A lunatic appears insensible, but his is, perhaps, the most alive of any mind to ridicule, and to the contemptibleness of his state. But he is, as I may say, unconsciously alive to it. He does not acknowledge his own feelings, because his mind is deeply engrossed in painful and excruciating conflicts; he is already troubled by a thousand horrible and fanciful ideas of danger; the victim of inward and preternatural sarcasm, contumely, and derision. But he acts strangely, from what he suffers unacknowledged and not understood by himself. If indeed,

---

124   Such lines demonstrate why it was not difficult to determine Perceval's identity upon publication, as the assassination of his father would have been infamous.

125   "Nervous patient" was a common euphemism, especially for upper-class patients whose family would not have wanted them associated with the "mad-house."

he were in quiet, peaceful circumstances, if he were secure he might find his mind reflect to his conscience perfectly, what the trouble occasioned by internal and external alarm prevents him noting; but the opposite is his position.

Though all men in the world are daily acting more or less from these unacknowledged sensations, I shall not be understood without mentioning an example. Whenever I went out to walk, on leaving the common room and turning round to the left into the passage, I had to pass by the door of the housekeeper's room, before I reached the hall door. Into this room I often ran from my keeper at the command of one or other of the spirits, and began to admire the maid's work-baskets, and similar objects which, though trifling, appeared to me so simple, neat, and beautiful. I used often to wonder at myself, and to be surprised, that what formerly I passed over with neglect, now so greatly attracted me. When I was in a great measure recovered from my delusions, and in better health, keeping also a constant and minute watch and control over my actions, and observing the causes of them, I went out, one day, walking as usual, when on passing the door of that room, I observed the shadows and voices of persons entering the hall door on the right. I ran immediately, as formerly, into the housekeeper's room, unable to check the impulse. I recollected myself, however, and then recognised that it was acute sensitiveness or shyness; the consciousness of my being unfit for the eye of man to look upon, that caused me to rush into the servants' apartments, with whom I was in some degree familiarized, rather than meet the gaze of a stranger. I said instantly to myself "then the physician is unconscious that we have any feeling; and is mistaken in his system." I felt the hopelessness of my situation, at the same time that I saw how necessary seclusion was for my happiness and peace of mind, to preserve me from acts of folly.

From what I state, it will be obvious how improper for many patients any exposure, or any conduct likely to draw attention on them in particular must be. Nature tells a man, who has any great grief, to be for a time secluded. Nature makes a man, sensible of any great infirmity, seek retirement, still more under such an awful infliction as insanity, when from the proud station of a reasonable being, he is degraded below the beasts of the field: fallen from his throne; bereft of his dominion. Nature, however, comes not into any part of the doctor's plans, but self-interest. He does not consider what is the sanest treatment for the sufferers, but what will attract most customers. They see the patients apparently unconscious to the shame of their situation; and that conduct, which really proceeds from an unacknowl-edged sense of it, they look upon as a sign of the specific disease they labour under. They act then according to that they find, instead of reflecting that want of sense is probably part of the disease, and that it is their duty *to restore a sense* of propriety by more regard on their part, not to harden the feelings by constant exposure. I may apply the same remarks to the custom of walking me about the grounds, where I met the carriages of the visitors, and others about the farm-houses, and subsequently, with a string of patients through the villages: what could be more painful to a man of any feeling? what could be more dangerous if you wished to restore good-feeling? what more cruel if it was the design to probe the feelings, through a heart already broken down, and benumbed by disease and affliction?

I may be wrong, but I cannot help suspecting that it was the key to Dr. F.'s system to probe the feelings; if not, why put such brutal questions? why take the patients by surprise at the visit of relations? why expose them in public to receive private communications? why insult them and degrade them in every circumstance of domestic life, toilette, meals, couch, &c. &c.; besides on one occasion, when I remarked to Marshall that the boots were not very well cleaned, he replied with his strong nasal twang, "they'll be better when you get out, d'ye see."

When I began to make remonstrances with my family, I complained of the absurdity of their having allowed me to be exposed in this manner, at the same time that the professed object of my being detained so far from home, was the desire pretended for *my* retirement, to save *my* feelings in not meeting my friends. I alluded, amongst other facts, to my having been allowed and encouraged to go out to play at cricket, with strange gentlemen of the neighbourhood, whilst yet hallooing out, and acting under the wildest delusions. And when the propriety of my being in retirement was again recurred to as an argument, to prevent my confinement in London, or in a neighbourhood where I hoped to meet those who would truly befriend me, since my relations on pretence of duty, delicacy, or decency, abandoned me to the malice and economy of the doctor, I replied, that such an argument was sheer mockery; that not my pride, not my delicacy, not my modesty were being consulted, not my care for privacy, but my family's desire to hide me; for otherwise they would make my privacy effectual by placing me in a private family as I required;[126] and whether was it better to have my griefs and infirmities exposed to friends who would

---

126 Single-patient care was a popular alternative to the private asylum for wealthy patients—Perceval advocated strongly for this kind of care, especially once he felt he had returned to sanity.

enter into my feelings, respect, pity, and protect me, or to the strange tenantry, strange household, strange patients, and strange visitors of a doctor perfectly unknown to me, except through his stupid inhumanity.

O sirs! the conduct I have had to endure, the gauntlet I have had to run through was dreadful; but it cannot be remedied now; when my mind recurs to it, it is too great to be resented articulately.

I desired my family to order Dr. F. to let me walk nowhere but in his kitchen garden, the place least liable to the intrusion of strangers, and that I might be alone. This was attended to; and I am thankful it was, otherwise I might never have been restored to LIBERTY.*[127]

---

127 [Perceval's footnote] *One afternoon, a thunderstorm came on whilst we were in the field at cricket; my spirits were then as usual puzzling me, when suddenly a rattling peal of thunder shook the vault of the heavens, to my ears it articulated the most terrible imprecations, and I stood mute with astonishment, expecting almost to be struck to the earth by the lightning, and doubting whether to attribute my being spared to the mercy and long suffering of God, or to the infinite counsels of his wrath reserving me for greater damnation. A passage of scripture has since been brought to my mind, when a voice came from heaven, but some said it thundered.*

CHAPTER XXVI

MY RECOVERY WAS VERY GRADUAL, but its periods remarkable. Three times my spirits prophesied to me, that a great change would take place in my situation. I expected a marvel, but the change took place in me, by natural causes, altering my apparent relationship to the persons around me. I had been continually haunted by the idea, that the sufferings I saw or fancied others enduring, were endured for me, and that it was my duty to try to partake in them or to alleviate them, or to perform some act of duty, for my neglect of which they were punished in my stead. For instance, when one day I saw the young clergyman, Mr. J. fastened opposite to me in a niche, by an iron manacle to the wall; *in great agitation I prayed the servant* not to do so, but to put it on me instead. For he had been kind to me, and I heard the spirits say or sing to me, "Mr. J. is manacled for you." But after one of the prophecies mentioned above, I began to hear these words added to the message of the spirits, Mr. J. is manacled, or suffocating, or whatever it might be, for you; to meditate on and reflect on too, or to think on with grief and contrition too, and the like. Then I knew that I had been deceived; and my mind received quiet. I was relieved from the oppression that I was continually causing the misery of others by my misdemeanours, and from the harass of being always called upon to perform some hazardous duty in order to relieve them. I began to hesitate before I acted, waiting on any appeal from a spirit, to hear if no interpretation or additional sentence explained the first. I joked inwardly at the absurdity of my delusions. By this a great alteration took place in my mind. Objects began to stand around me in a new light. I began to be less ready to give up the dictates of common sense, to the injunctions of invisible agents. At another time, my spirits began singing to me in this strain. "You are in a lunatic asylum, if you will"—"if not, you are in," &c. &c. "That is Samuel Hobbs if you will—if not, it is Herminet Herbert," &c. &c. &c. But I had been so long deceived by my spirits that now I did not believe them when they spoke truth. However, by listening and finding that the patients called him Samuel Hobbs, and by other accidents, I discovered at last that I was yet on earth, in natural, although very painful, circumstances in a madhouse. My delusions being thus very much abolished, I soon after got liberty of limb during the day-time.

Then new delusions succeeded those that were dissipated. I was on earth, it was true, in England and in a lunatic asylum; but I understood that it was the law of the land, that those lunatics who after a certain trial did not recover should be made away with, in order to spare the country the expense of maintaining them. I was still a disobedient angel whom the Lord had made pass for a lunatic in order to preserve me. But I was watched with jealousy. Several times my spirits indicated to me a gentleman who was, I afterwards discovered, a patient in another ward, as the Chancellor of the Exchequer.[128] He had come down purposely to examine and report upon my case. He was not the only person I dignified with title and office. Before that, when the magistrates paid their first visit, I imagined that one was the Lord Eldon, the other Mr. Goulburn, and a third my mother's attorney.[129] They had come to look after me, both out of respect to my father, and from the peculiar interest that my case excited. But, when I came to see my delusions, I received these grave old useless gentlemen with bursts of laughter, both at their demeanour, and at the absurdity of my deception. I shook off the greatest part of my delusions a short time before the riots at Bristol.

About this time, one of my brothers came to see me. I did not receive him very kindly. I was beginning to suspect that my family had behaved ill to me, though unable to express myself, or to arrange my ideas. There was an inquisitiveness also in my brother's manner which I did not think becoming, accompanied with the same tone of suspicion I had observed in the Mr. F—s', which wounded my feelings and aroused my pride. During our conversation, my brother asked me why I spoke with my mouth shut, and whether I had been used to do so. I did not understand the question, but on his repeating it, I put my hand up to my mouth when speaking, and to my surprise found that whilst I spoke I kept my teeth close together. Soon after, he noticed my

---

128 Finance minister.

129 Mr Goulburn is likely Henry Goulburn, the Chancellor of the Exchequer between 1828-30. Lord Eldon had been Lord Chancellor of the United Kingdom until 1827. The Lord Chancellor is appointed by the monarch as a highly ranked cabinet member with responsibility for the courts. The Lord Chancellor also had purview over those wealthy lunatics who lost power to dispose of their own affairs—so called "chancery lunatics." Chancery lunatics could request extraordinarily expensive, and often very public, trials to establish their sanity.

hair was cut very close and cropped in front, but long and full behind. I was not aware of that either until he drew my attention to it. He asked me if I liked it being cut so. I said to myself, if he is such a fool as to ask such a question, I am a fool to talk with him seriously; but I suspected that this was a part of the insulting system I had been submitted to, and that my brother asked me merely to try if I resented it. The absurdity of such a system, whoever imagined it, cannot be better evidenced than by my never having noticed the affront; and the result of it, when I noticed it, was, that I resolved to show no resentment, whatever I might feel. I then proposed taking a walk with my brother, to show him a view over to Bristol, which I admired very much. The attendant followed us.

On returning, my brother went up with me to see my bed-room. He asked me also if I should like to see an aunt and a cousin, who were interested about me. I replied unfortunately, that I thought it would be of no use. I felt that I should only be grieving them, and that they could not find out for me the clue to those puzzling inspirations which troubled my mind. But their coming would no doubt have cheered and enlivened me, and as they both loved me, they might either have felt and remedied the impropriety of my situation, or have taken me home with them upon trial, for I was then perfectly inoffensive. In that case ease, quiet, and security would have rapidly effectuated my cure.

The same evening I dined with my brother at Dr. F's. The conversation turned on Mr. Irving, and other topics: I did not feel satisfied with the style of those who took part in it. I heard all that was said; but I was conversing chiefly with my spirits. At one time they were teazing me about the manner in which I was to eat or leave my potatoes, and at last, not being able to please myself or them, I threw down my knife and fork on the plate: this attracted a moment's observation. Mr. F. F. said a few silly words in joke, and I resumed my tranquillity and gentleness. Next morning, being Sunday, I saw my brother again in Mr. F. F.'s company after church for about half an hour, on the lawn by the old doctor's house. I behaved very coolly, and I suppose he felt no encouragement to see me again. On Monday morning, he took leave of me at the hall door of the madhouse, and mounted one of the doctor's horses to ride into Bristol. He is no great horseman, and I re-entered the prison I was confined to with Samuel Hobbs, holding my arm, and laughing and quizzing at his want of jockeyship.

I was sensible to the impertinence of this familiarity, but my feelings of resentment against my family made it in some sense not unpleasing, particularly as I thought there was an expression of sympathy in the man's countenance, and of disappointment at the result of my brother's visit. They have not touched the right string, he seemed to say, they have been too dull to guess the secret. To resent familiarity, however, on the part of the domestics, was to break through at once the whole system of polite education I had been submitted to. This man had walked arm in arm with me, recited Shakspeare to me, sang songs, trifled, fooled with me. His language was neither restrained by reverence or decency, and often he swore. He always talked in an insolent radical manner of the gentry. My spirits often desired me to rebuke him, when I was shocked at his oaths and language. But I refused; for, I replied, if these offences are really rebuke-worthy, I will keep my rebukes for those who really need them; not for those who sin designedly, to tempt me from curiosity, or from some other motive.

Besides, I used to reply, if this is the Lord Jesus Christ, he cannot really sin, and I will not expose my want of faith and stupidity to ridicule and mockery by rebuking that, which since the universal redemption I have been informed of, is no more rebuke-worthy. But when I had recovered a sounder understanding, I knew that this man was substantially and indeed Samuel Hobbs, the servant of a doctor of lunatics, whatever might be his spiritual character. It fell out one afternoon, about the time of the Bristol riots, when the speech of our servants became very licentious, and the threats of what was to be done to the gentry very wondrous, and yet alarming, that he was sitting with his back towards the table, his feet upon the fender, and his pipe in his mouth, and slandering many great men, and the gentry generally. I then felt for my companion, Captain P. whom my spirits had called my spirit of family pride; and when at last he fell foul of the Duke of Wellington, I told him to hold his tongue, and to mind his own business; that the Duke of Wellington was a greater man than he or I were ever likely to be; and that till we could imitate his great actions, we might make allowance for his slight faults.[130] After this, I never heard Samuel Hobbs speak disrespectfully of the nobility again. Whether or no he was ashamed of being rebuked by a madman, he acknowledged the justice of this reproof.

No doubt Dr. F. and others will express their surprise on hearing these facts, and say they disown them to be, and

---

130   As a member of the upper classes, Perceval would have been very nervous about the kinds of revolutionary sentiments behind the Bristol Riots. Notably, his speech in defense of Wellington stands in contradiction to his earlier critique of Wellington, whose politics he suggested drove him from the Tory party and the military. This suggests his allegiance to class above party.

ask why they were not complained of. I reply, would it not have been a sensible and a reasonable course to pursue, to complain of these things? Were not we confined because we were deranged in our reason, and bereft of our senses? Am not I right then in saying that the world, in their treatment of lunatics, are as insane as the lunatic himself, inasmuch as they expect from one expressly devoid of reason, the conduct of a reasonable being. Again, supposing that by chance one or two of the lunatics acknowledge the impropriety of the conduct that passes round them, yet, *if their moral sense is not blunted to the enormity of it*, by their habitual degradation as well as by disease, why should they complain either to the magistrates or the doctor, when they do not know that such conduct is not connived at, when they know that whatever they say is looked upon with mistrust and suspicion, and that in either case they are left exposed to the malice and brutality of those whom they complain against; to whose evidence they may have to look also shortly for the recovery of their liberty.

Soon after liberty of limb had been restored to me, my mother, to whose exertions I owe, after all, whatever was likely to restore me to sound reason whilst under the care of Dr. F., begged that I might be allowed to work in his garden; this was indeed beneficial, as it gave me occupation and more privacy. Later in the year I was employed with two gentlemen and a keeper, to cut out a small path in the shrubbery. I was entrusted with the mattock and the spade. My spirits however teazed me so much, by contrary directions, that after repeated trials I threw them down, contenting myself to wheel the barrow, to pick up sticks, and to handle the bill-hook.[131] It was about the time of the Bristol riots.

---

131   A heavy chopping implement with a hooked end used for gardenwork.

The seditious conversation and tone of the servants, and their accounts of the state of mind of the peasantry, gave me great anxiety. The heavy dragoons[132] were quartered in the neighbourhood, and one day I saw a troop of them exercising their horses down the road. They talked loudly and swore. I augured ill of their trustworthiness and discipline from their conduct, and throwing down the sticks I had been collecting, I rushed into the thicket in tears, exclaiming, "oh! my country, oh! my country." Then my spirits checked me; I began to sing a psalm, and was beguiled by my delusions. At that time, I longed to see a train of artillery coming down the road, and looked for it daily; for I knew that they would keep order; but the government then acted the part of madmen if not worse. The night the city was on fire, Hobbs and Poole came into my bed-room to see the flames; I was tied in bed; Poole proposed to untie me, that I might see it; but Hobbs replied, "Oh! no, no, he will only be playing his tricks."

One day whilst working in this plantation, the string of patients passed us on their way home. Hobbs took me by the arm and laughed saying, "come let us see what you have been doing, they say you do nothing but pick up the sticks like an old woman." He came at last to the bundles I had collected to light his fire; he seemed to reflect, and was silent. Another day, old Benevolence presented me with a fine nettle, in white bloom which he had gathered in a hedge, and told me it was a green house plant. The size made me hesitate for a moment, but I saw immediately it was a joke. Then my behaviour in the asylum struck me in its true light; the scales fell from my eyes.[133] I knew that I was looked upon

---

132 Cavalry soldiers with firearms.

133 A reference to Acts 9:18, when "something like scales" fell off the eyes of

as a child; what, thought I, you take me for a child, for a fool! but you do not know what has made me so! On another occasion whilst amusing myself with the bill-hook, an old clergyman came to me to request me to yield it up to him: I said, quietly, "No! I like to use it myself;" he went up to the keeper, and I saw them laughing heartily. I reflected then on what I had spoken, and could not help laughing myself, whilst I walked up to him and gave him the bill hook.

We were not the only gulls; Dr. F. had in his premises, on the lawn before the house, four or five fed, which had been brought from the sea.[134] They strayed across the field into the plantation in which I was employed, and I drove them back with my pocket handkerchief. It was the first time I was trusted alone. A female came out and thanked me; then the sight of a female at all beautiful, was enchanting to me.

I now began to recover my reflection rapidly, and to make observations upon characters and persons around me. I met the doctor who had bled me in the temporal artery, when going out one day at the hall door. Some of my spirits desired me to resent the manner in which this operation had been performed, without my permission, and in a brutal way; and I do to this day; but, others desired me to forgive him. These on the whole prevailed. I shook hands with him to show him that I bore him no ill-will; and on his alluding to my state, I said, "Oh! sir, I have been in a dream, a fearful dream, but it is gone now."

I had asked Mr. F. F. for a pocket-book in order to know the date, and to keep memoranda. He gave it me one

---

Saul, signifying both the return of his physical sight and his recognition that Jesus was the messiah.

134   Perceval appears to be playing with a double meaning of gull: gull as in the bird, and gull as in gullible or foolish person.

day out of a gig, whilst I was employed in the shrubbery: I vaulted over a gate to receive it. I had told him before this, that I should make my escape if I could, that I might not be accused of being guilty of a breach of trust if I ran away. He remarked, I see you are active enough to attempt your threatened escape, but I suppose you do not really mean it. I replied, I really did. So simple was I, and so resolved. I should say that by this time my mind had arrived from a state of imbecility and infancy, through a state of childishness, to the simplicity of boyhood; open and undisguised, and designing adventures, without calculating its strength.

Later in the year my imagination began to reflect the most divine and beautiful figures, in all kind of lascivious and wanton combination; until then my mind had been as chaste as it was free from malice. Now I saw these angelic forms, more beautiful than pictures, because they changed their attitudes, and sported in action. My spirits however told me that I had been looking on these scenes all the time that I was in the mad-house, that that was what they meant by heavenly places, and when I reminded them that I never had been able to get to heavenly places, they said that was my fault; that my spirit had been there, and that they had often desired me to come up there in one spirit or another; but that they could not help it if my spirit only came, and I chose to remain behind. With these visions I heard voices, reconciling me to the sight of, and desiring me to become a partaker in the lewd acts I saw committing; obliterating my disgust, and all sense of guilty shame, and substituting a purer feeling of delicate submission and modest consent. The holiness of the images purified the imagery of all that was revolting; and if my spirit refused to acknowledge the pleasure I took in contemplating these scenes and actions, and the desire I had to partake in them, then I was made to imagine as if in spirit I was forced to submit to the same, with every accompaniment of violence, insult, degradation, and sarcasm, as a puritanical and ungrateful hypocrite; undeserving of my Heavenly Father's love, in thus revealing his goodness to me, and unveiling his true nature, of which the world were ignorant, and kept in ignorance by him, through their hypocrisies, and malice, and envy one towards the other.

CHAPTER XXVII

I WILL NOW TURN to the conduct and treatment of my wretched companions in confinement, and in affliction. I will begin with the oldest and most noisy of them all. A grey haired, bald headed, thin old gentleman, whom I first called Dr. F., and then my uncle, Mr. D., whose name also he bore. He was a solicitor or an attorney, he wore an old-fashioned, long skirted, square-cut black coat, and a broad brimmed hat, and when in good health, he was very respectable in appearance. He was usually very red in the face, idiotic, noisy, jabbering sentences of Virgil, Horace, English, &c., &c., occasionally applying them with a hidden meaning. He would halloo, strike the others in sport, and was altogether mischievous and troublesome. He often scratched his head till it was quite sore in many places; once he baptized me on my seat, whilst fastened up, with a mug of beer: once he threw brickbats[135] at me. This was the gentleman my arm slapped in the face after he had struck me a blow at tea. He was usually to be seen in a room upstairs, with his red wild face staring through the blinds; here he was confined

---

135 Lumps of brick.

alone. When I began to walk about the yard, he would put his arm round my shoulder, ask me to walk with him, seize me by the right ear, and pulling it ask me, "Is that the ear Dr. L. opened for you?" Occasionally he pinched the wounded ear, but more gently. He did it to arouse me. He would ask me questions on Latin poetry;—I suspect it was he that hid the Bible. When he walked out with us, I observed that at stated distances he picked up a large stone, and carrying it a little way, threw it into one place, till at last there was a pretty large heap of stones collected at one of these stations. When I was recovering, he confided to me part of his story by snatches, under a chaos of confused sentences, allusions, and quotations. He told me he had been a lawyer, practising on the western circuit; that he had written a letter with a benevolent intention, at the time of my father's death, relating to my family. He inquired into circumstances connected with his views in that letter, his ideas were rational and distinct on the subject; though he could hardly speak three sentences coherently; like the under current of a stream, which remains clear and steady in its course, though broken at the surface and at the banks into a thousand eddies, and by a thousand waves. There was another subject preyed upon his mind, connected with his conduct at the Taunton assizes,[136] where it appeared there was danger of the rescue of certain prisoners, and he had taken an active part; he appeared to be scrupulous about his conduct having been correct, and he mingled also allusions to his daughter; but there his mind failed him; he could not explain himself directly. Another day he spoke of my treatment by the servants. He told me he thought I had been

---

136   Assizes were legal proceedings heard by judges on a regional circuit. Taunton is in the south-west of England, about fifty miles from Bristol.

illtreated, and that the behaviour of the servants was very bad. I replied, that I did not think it was intentional: he said, "I do," and then ran off on other subjects, as if afraid to say too much. He was more than seventy years of age, and I thought it a sad thing to see an old man in so great affliction, who had been so respectable, confined in such circumstances, and I wondered at the want of feeling of Dr. F., who was himself an old man.

I will mention next, Captain ——, the most prominent character in the room. My spirits desired me to call him Executioner, and Patience. He was of a brown complexion, with dark glossy hair; he had lost one leg, and besides had a withered arm, the sleeve of which was fastened to the breast of a blue surtout coat:[137] he had a cork leg. He stood for one half the year at the end of the room facing the window, sitting down only at meals, and never leaving the room except to be shaved, or to go to bed, and once in the forenoon. He was usually silent, but occasionally cried aloud strange words; "Bruim!" &c.; or spoke a few disjointed sentences, in which he anathematized the Duke of York, and Sir Herbert Taylor,[138] or abused the servants. He had dark penetrating expressive eyes. A newspaper was often brought to him, which sometimes he tore up, sometimes he allowed to be read in the room. He often complained aloud of the thickness of the bread and butter at breakfast and at tea. I remarked that there was usually one slice of bread and butter twice the thickness of all the rest, put on his plate. This is one of the reasons which make me suspect that the patient's feelings were often provoked designedly, either through

---

137 Overcoat.

138 Readers may recall that it was to the Duke of York and Sir Herbert Taylor that Perceval owed his military commission.

the impertinent jocularity of the keepers, or through the mistaken quackery of the doctor. One forenoon about the middle of the year, a chair was brought in, and fastened below by an iron chain to the wall, and two servants seized this gentleman and forced him violently to sit down upon it. After that he remained seated in one position the rest of the year. He reminded me very much of the Brahmins[139] I have read of, who imagine that they devote themselves to God in keeping one attitude all their lives. When the chair and the iron chain were brought in, I was very much frightened; I was then fastened up, and I thought he was going to be tortured for me. I was to have had my stomach squeezed between the chain and the floor, because I was such a glutton, and refused nothing for the sake of any spirit, but in pity for me. Patience had undertaken to endure it for me. I hallooed out to spare him, and was greatly excited. I saw him forced on the seat, and not under the chain. Then the spirits told me that he had endured it, but that they would not let me see it, they had hidden it from my eyes. Perhaps nothing can prove more strongly the power of my delusions, than that I gave credit to this absurd explanation. The reasons were that I believed in the tale of the destruction of Sodom and Gomorrah, when the eyes of a whole mob were blinded so that they could not find Lot's door! I conjectured that Jesus had escaped through the midst of the people by being rendered invisible to them: and I had myself been often perplexed by seeing persons who were not around me, instead of persons who were: by seeing words in books that were not printed there, and by other illusions. There was nothing else striking in the demeanour of Captain ———, but that he occasionally in manner and in speech, exhibited

139   Hindu priests.

his resentment of the disrespectful conduct of the servants.

Mr. N——, my spirits called Mr. Fazakerley, and my spirit of delicacy and contrition. He was a short, thin, sharp featured man, with light grey eyes, a mouth always pursed with sardonic smiles, a head partly bald and partly grey. He carried his hands usually in his waistcoat or trouser pockets; walked with a nonchalant obstinate air, and with an awkward gait, halting on one leg. He was a man of pride. He sat usually in one chair by the fireplace, his elbow leaning on a table, and never spoke to any around him; once or twice only I heard him ask a question, and give directions to the servants, who treated him with decorum. Two or three times a day he rose from his chair and went into the yard, where he stood with his head raised up, his hands on his hips, his face wearing the appearance of choking, and cried aloud, "I take my oath before God, &c. &c. &c., that I *am* the Duke of Somerset, and that I give and bequeath all my jewels, large possessions, &c. &c., to his majesty and his heirs for ever. So help me God. Amen!" When I went into the yard at liberty, the spirits desired me also to take his position, and to cry out in like manner; "I am the lost hope of a noble family;" but after attempting it three or four times, I shrunk from so exposing my feelings, and my situation. Then my spirits said, cry out, "God save the king," or any thing you like, but you must suffocate. Mr. Fazakerley suffocates himself in this position, you must do the same. I took this direction literally, and I tried to sing the words, and at the same time choke myself. And I conceived myself a hypocrite because I could not perform an impossibility; which however perhaps, I had no intention of performing sincerely. Not succeeding in my attempt to suffocate, or in understanding the directions of the spirits who offered to teach me, and feeling the exposure of my situation, I used to stand in that place the greater part of the morning and of the afternoon. In the autumn when I had left this off, Hobbs showed me that part of the privet hedge, behind which I stood, saying, "look here, what you have done;" it was literally stripped of its leaves, yet I was not aware of having plucked them; this will show the nervous state in which I had been, and how great was my mental agony. I do not know what Mr. Fazakerley thought, but I rather think my conduct cured him of his folly, or diminished the exhibition of it. Once always in the afternoon Mr. Fazakerley rose and marching towards the cupboard near which I was confined, took out of it a cup which he filled from a can of water, left in the room after dinner. My spirits desired me repeatedly to ask him for a cup of cold water also, but he never gave me one; but he whom I called Affection, did.

This was a Rev. Mr. J., a clergyman from Devonshire, a tall sallow complexioned man, with light hair, a firm, but kind and gentle, though vacant countenance, somewhat slovenly. The agony of his features was often very great. He made observations aloud, often of a spiritual nature, not very delicate in language, sometimes reasoning on the anomalous character of the servants, as if arguing with himself what was his proper line of conduct towards them, occasionally replying in a very loud tone to the remarks of another patient. He stamped also with one foot, with a remarkably earnest expression of countenance at the same time. He was often treated violently, and manacled to the seat opposite to me. I never could tell why, for I never saw him offer violence to any one, except late in the year, when he had a quarrel with an impertinent young man, and they scuffled. He bore the illtreatment of the servants with a most provokingly calm superiority of humour. It was this gentleman who was so agitated, when they were forcing the meat down my throat. He was repeatedly pushed out of the room for his noise. I heard him once reasoning aloud on the sacrament, and made a few observations to him. He addressed me several times by name, always in an earnest and friendly manner, and now and then turned away again laughing, as much as to say, this young man does not want preaching or wisdom, he wants to be at fun and mockery all the day through. My spirits called him my cousin ———'s, spirit of family affection, also that he was my cousin, the most affectionate of my relations and friends, also when I desired them to show me St. John the Apostle, they directed me to look on him, whilst they told me that I was like to St. Paul or to St. Peter.

One afternoon in the summer time, I staid in doors with other patients, whilst the rest went out walking; when they came in, after Hobbs had locked the door, I was standing by the fire-place, and Mr. J. was passing along the other side of the table towards the yard; he took off his hat and put it on the table, making some observations aloud. Hobbs who had come near me on my side of the table, spoke sharply to him and lifted a cane he had in his hand. Mr. J. replied, pray who are you; then offering his arm said, you may strike me if you will. Hobbs struck him three or four sharp cuts over the arm across the table. Mr. J. smiled contemptuously at him, stamped with his foot, put his hat on his head, and passed out of the room. Had I been a little more in my senses, I should probably have thrashed the servant.

The gross want of respect to situation, rank, character, or profession, manifested by these men on all occasions, is shocking to the imagination, and revolting to reflection; and also, that whilst a lunatic is exposed to immediate and unsparing chastisement from them, for any ebullition of frenzy; he may be tempted to acts of violence repeatedly, both in self-defence, and in common justice to others; which nevertheless, by the ignorant and shuffling magistrate who visit him, would be infallibly perverted into a proof of his continued insanity, upon the report of those who are most interested to distort facts to detain him, and to revenge themselves upon him for his noble and spirited resistance, and uncompromising representations. The very acts of impatience and impetuosity which gave me self-confidence and hope, and assured me I was returning to my sound senses, too sound to be liked by those feeding on my supineness and imbecility; the very acts which I hailed in my fellow-prisoners as symptoms of restored life, and of gallant, though God knows, imprudent resentment of galling mockery, insult, and oppression, were looked upon, and held up by my doctor to the keepers as the signs of mania; the very disorder for which I was to be detained. But that which my mind found more terrible, was that whilst temptations to violence should have been removed from me, on account of my express state, we were continually provoked to use violence, with justice and honour to human nature; the result of which however, might have been fatal to those who excited our acts, and then have consigned the unfortunate perpetrator of them to be entombed for life in a madhouse; as far at least probably as any inquiry before a jury would have availed him, and certainly if he had property to pay the doctor well for keeping him.

One morning when Mr. J. had asserted that he had done nothing to deserve confinement, Samuel Hobbs replied, "how can you say so sir, didn't I come to fetch you, and when I came hadn't you kicked through your brother's door, and weren't they afraid to keep you in the house, and you would not go out of it." I do not know if these are sufficient grounds for shutting a man up in a madhouse, but Samuel Hobbs thought so, and he got his bread by it.

Mr. W—— was an old gentleman, about sixty years of age, bald-headed, of short stature, rather stout, an aquiline nose, and silly smiling countenance. He was the first of the patients who tried to enter into conversation with me, and with whom I endeavoured to exchange any reasonable remarks. I called him Mr. Simplicity. He used to stand by me when fastened upon my wooden seat in the niche, leaning slightly against the wall with his hands in his pockets, jabbering with an appearance of great self-complacency a great many unconnected sentences, mentioning my name, alluding to my father in a tone of surprise and encouragement, sometimes addressing to me appeals against the conduct of the servants. He was an Irishman, and a quaker; he had been partner and coheir in a bank at —— in Ireland, and had run away from the bank at the death of his father or of one of the proprietors, on account of his fears of being made liable for the overdrawing or speculations of a relation and copartner. He had been secured, and since that time for many long years confined in this madhouse. I collected these facts from his own lips, after painful and repeated attention to his wanderings; sometimes interrupting him, sometimes leading him back. I can give but a faint idea of the want of connexion of subjects betrayed by his conversation. He would speak thus: "yes, sir, yes, sir. Lord K. was a very good man, a very good man! Do you know Lord —— sir, he was Lord Lieutenant in my time. Yes, sir, and Mr. ——, and Mr. ——, the same as brought in the bill for emancipating the Roman Catholics, you know sir; my father was at that time head of the firm. Sallust, you know Sallust, sir, one of the Roman authors, he kept a bank at ——, county of Limerick.[140] S—— and Co. My father knew the duke of Richmond very well. Yes, sir, it was a very respectable firm. Mr. ——'s, son in a madhouse! they say he's not mad but only pretends to be so. Yes, sir, he was an old man. We are quakers. That rascal Hobbs threatens to put the manacles on me (here he used to seize his wrist, tremble, and speak very loud and fluently), he threatens to strike me, sir; I wonder if Dr. F. knows of it. Dublin, yes, Dublin is a very fine town. So when my father died I suspected it was not all right, you see, sir, I ran away. There was a great disturbance in Cork, and Mr. —— was member for the county; they wanted to make me liable; so I thought it better to run away. There's a great sum owing to me now. I spoke to Dr. F. about it; I asked for some writing paper, but Hobbs takes it all away, he takes every thing away from me, sir. The doctors say that my case is that of pavor lymphaticus, pavor lymphaticus,[141] sir."

And so it was, poor old gentleman, for at the slightest appearance of menace from any of the patients or servants, he called out lustily, took his hands out of his pockets and stretched them out trembling from head to foot, though a stout man. At the latter end of the year I was disgusted by seeing Marshall seize him on two or three occasions by the collar of the coat and throw him on the back upon the floor; it was in sport, but improper and rude sport from one old man to another, and from the servant and keeper of lunatic patients; to a patient under lymphaticus pavor. This old man was quiet and timid like a child. I soon found out that there was some foundation for his complaints against Samuel

---

140 Gaius Sallustius Crispus, a first-century BCE Roman historian.

141 Latin: frantic panic.

Hobbs. He was generally allowed after breakfast to go up to his bed-room to read, and it was amusing even there to see him eagerly steal away delighted to get out of reach of danger, but Hobbs often stopped him in his flight, saying, "hallo, Mr. —— where are you going to, sir, you shall not go up." Or after *hearing him* rating him on the stairs in a loud voice, he brought him down again; whether from caprice or not I cannot tell. I found when I was allowed to be upstairs myself, that the old man studied Sallust, and wanted me to construe to him some passages; this accounted for the mention of that author. Having been at Dublin, I often tried to talk with him of that city, for there was no one else cared to know what he was gabbling about.

In the autumn, Captain W. a young Irish gentleman, an officer in the line, having been brought to the house, made jest of poor Mr. Simplicity, threatening to throw things at him, to strike him, &c. &c. Captain W. read a great deal in the Prayer book. This gave me hopes of reasoning with him on the impropriety of his conduct: besides that, he was really a gentleman. But to my astonishment and amusement he argued quietly and in sober seriousness. I am sure he was sent to me by God Almighty to keep me from melancholy, I should die in such a stupid place if I had not him to make fun of. My spirits called this old gentleman like many others, Mr. Fitzherbert: he was but a slovenly old fellow standing always with his hands in his breeches pockets, a posture for the hands however not unusual or surprising in a house where we were all devoted to idleness and sloth.

Beyond him, on my left hand side, sat a little, thin, withered, yellow faced man, sprucely dressed, with a well brushed blue coat and brass buttons, neat frill, waistcoat, and drab trousers, white stockings, and shoes, his grey head neatly combed, his legs uncrossed before him, his white handkerchief spread on his knees, and his hands on his thighs. My spirits called him Decency; he occupied this seat morning and afternoon invariably, except when out walking or at meals, when he took a turn or two up and down one side of the yard. He was a Dr. S———. I heard that he had been confined for twenty years, and had fought a duel. He was a quiet, silent, inoffensive man. I seldom heard him speak at all. Once only he spoke to me in the autumn, in a very squeaking voice when he showed me a withering leaf, and told me the mottled colours on it reminded him of an apple. One day I saw him go up stairs with a clean pair of blinds, I presume to fasten before his window; unfortunately Hobbs was in the way, caught him, made him come back, and snatched the blinds out of his hands, and rated him, saying, "I told you you should not go up, I'll take the blinds and throw them to the devil."

By the side of Mr. Decency, sat Captain P., another of the numerous family of Fitzherbert, that the spirits pointed out to me. When at last I asked what was the meaning of that name, and how so many came to bear it who had no relationship to each other, they replied, that Fitzherbert meant son of Herbert, and that these being spiritual bodies, were all sons of the almighty Herminet Herbert, whom I had seen in the three persons of the trinity; Herminet Herbert, God Almighty; Herminet Herbert, Jesus Christ; and Herminet Herbert, the Holy Ghost; and also in Herminet Herbert, the Trinity in Unity; and that the name of Herbert, signified from the German, Lord of Hell.[142] The Mr. Fitzherbert in question, was my spirit of family pride, and gentlemanly decorum. He was the most gentlemanly and courteous

---

142   See note 64.

individual in the room; tall, well made, with dark hair and eye brows, good features, and a countenance inclined to ruddiness, always clean and neat, without affectation. For a long time his actions served as signs to me. He usually occupied the same seat in the room, occasionally leaving it to play at cards: he seemed to feel his situation very acutely; often appeared to labour with great internal struggles, when he muttered deep in his throat something that seemed to be a quotation from a tragedy of a very bloody import, leaning forward at the same time, and wringing and turning his hands clasped within each other. It was he who stated to me the reason of his silence, for he scarcely ever spoke. I saw Hobbs once asking him to read a letter for him. The young doctor told me he laboured under certain delusions similar to mine.

At dinner, a Captain W. usually sat at the bottom of the table. He was also a Mr. Fitzherbert, my spirit of joviality, and of joviality in contrition. He was a short, stout, red faced, in happier circumstances I might have said, jolly looking man; quiet, mild, inoffensive in his manners, silent like the rest. That which particularly characterized him, was his being constantly in the yard, where he walked up and down, generally not under cover, and in all weather, unless it literally poured with rain. I thought this a symptom of derangement, but when I came to myself and spoke to him, he told me that he did it to be alone, he did not like the noise or the exposure of the common room. Besides this I may add, it was some occupation even to use the legs. This poor man had served in the Peninsula.[143] He answered any

---

143 The Iberian peninsula. It is not clear here what conflict if any he served in, though this might refer to the bloody Peninsular Wars of the early nineteenth century. British forces were led against France by the Duke of Wellington, mentioned by Perceval multiple times in this text.

question I put to him with perfect good sense, great deliber-
ation, and much agitation. I ceased to speak with him as he
never offered to begin conversation with me, and seeing him
apparently in the possession of all his faculties, I judged that
he might have reason for finding discourse painful, particularly with a stranger.

Here let me observe, if you want any proof of the madness as well as cruelty of applying a system such as this to
insane patients, where can you find one more perfect than
in the fact, that you drive them in self-defence to conduct
which in ordinary circumstances a man cannot fail to look
upon as a sign of an unsettled mind? You look upon the
unfortunate object of your pretended concern, and of your
occasional malevolence, with pity for irregularities and
extravagances, which however singular, however extravagant, are alas in him but too reasonable, through your
own unreasonableness; or putting him in circumstances
of extraordinary trial; do you expect from him, from him
whom you confine expressly for his weakness and defi-
ciency, an example of fortitude, a pattern of self-denial,
perhaps not to be found in the annals of human nature?
By reason of your own conduct, your judgment if honest
and scrupulous must be in ambiguity; for you can never tell
if the patient's eccentricities, are the symptoms of his disorder, or the result of antipathy to the new circumstances
in which you have placed him; and he, who is struggling
against the guilty tyranny and oppression of the doctor;
he who is dying daily to hope,—to life,—to the desire to
exercise those qualities of the mind, which for the sake of
woman endear a man to society, and society to man; he in
whose breast the seeds even of a divine nature, in spite of
your cruelty and contempt, rise to new life hourly, hourly

to be crushed and murdered, acknowledges amongst the crudest of his wrongs, and the hardest of his chains, that he must either tempt his nature to bear more than he can endure, or be condemned as insane, for actions and conduct arising from the faultiness of the conduct pursued towards him, the childishness of those who deal with him, and judge of him, forgetting his actual situation. To prefer walking in a cold drizzling rain, to sitting by a warm fire side, were folly, if your kindness were not coupled with that mockery, which makes the inclemency of the season and weather comparatively less cruel. To be silent and incommunicative is a singularity; but that singularity becomes reasonable, when a man is denied liberty of expression and action, and confined with perfect strangers, amidst those whose interest it is to suspect and pervert his ways; aware of that which you, enthroned in the conceit of a more sound understanding, are daily forgetting, that the weakness of his mind renders it peculiarly improper for him to open the secrets of his heart to men with whom he has even no acquaintance. To halloo, to bawl, to romp, to play the fool, are in ordinary life, signs of irregularity, but they become necessary to men placed in our position, to disguise or drown feelings for which we have no relief; too great for expression, too sacred for the prying eye of impertinent, impudent, and malevolent curiosity. I will be bound to say that the greatest part of the violence that occurs in lunatic asyla, is to be attributed to the conduct of those who are dealing with the disease, not to the disease itself; and that that behaviour which is usually pointed out by the doctor to the visitors as the symptoms of the complaint for which the patient is confined, is generally more or less a reasonable, and certainly a natural result, of that confinement, and its particular refinements in cruelty; for all have their select and exquisite moral and mental, if not bodily, tortures.

Captain W. was a man of a humble and humbled mind, susceptible, tender; the agitation of his feelings was often visible, in the trembling of his hands and arms. I used at first to kneel to him at night, to be saved from the tortures I thought prepared for me.

Mr. A. was a young man—fair, slight, quiet-mannered, stupid, good-tempered. He used to have novels lent to him, which he read usually whilst standing under the alcove in the yard—he put them by in the cupboard. I understood, on his remonstrating with me or another for taking the volume, that if he did not take care of them they would be taken away: so childish was our treatment, and so absurd. Was it in the first place more essential, that the only recreation and occupation by which a young gentleman could be called awhile from himself, and from contemplating his unfortunate position, should be secured to him; or that a novel in boards should be defaced—the price of which, after all, might be set down in the yearly accounts, in more perfect imitation of the private school system. Hobbs took away my books; but they were restored to me, when I complained of it, with an injunction to take care of them. I felt astonished and disgusted to be treated so like a child. But when I consider the propriety of the injunction, I ask, how were we to guard our effects, who had not so much as a drawer with a key to it, not even what boys have at school, a private locker. Oh! it is revolting to conceive this degrading treatment possible, and this in the midst of grown up Christian people, under a grown up old Quaker doctor, under the noses and eyes of big, bullying, grown up national church justices. It is revolting. It makes even this language, discreditable as it might be on other subjects—creditable, through the immensity of their folly, heedlessness, or "*supercherie*."[144] Yes, I say "supercherie," for the magistrates know well whether they are doing their duty, or affecting to do it. And if they reply, we act according to the statute; I answer, very well, gentlemen, then we'll look out for the making of some statute that will aid humanity, at the expense of your lauded indifference.

But again, to defend our property or trusts in a room full of madmen, where we were often left alone without the servants, and where we were confined ourselves with them, as too dangerous for society with all its understanding and force to cope with; too likely to invade the rights of others! He whose predisposition to violence was feared, exposed to collision in defence of his honour, and that amongst those shut up for their likelihood to invade honour!

Mr. A. conversed rationally, and joked with other patients. The spirits told me he was my brother D——, and my brother D.'s spirit of contrition. His countenance often wore the appearance of great lasciviousness. One day I recollect his standing by me with Mr. J., and quizzing me whilst manacled in the niche, when the other patients were out. He was an amiable young man, he went away in the autumn to Dublin, with Honesty, a kind and respectful servant. Long time before he went, the young doctor used to come and speak to him of his intended departure, and letters received. At last, to a question of Mr. J. as to whether he was going, he replied with a forced laugh, "that he did not believe he was going at all;" expressing himself contemptuously of the doctor—that he only came to sift him, and to pry into his feelings. Young Mr. J. replied quietly, "do you think so, I

144　Foul play.

think you are going." "I don't," replied Mr. A., and resumed the novel he was reading.

Captain ———, the gentleman whom my spirits called "the Lord Jehovah supremely omnipotent, the Trinity in unity," incorporate under the form of Mr. Waldong, Benevolence, &c. was a stout, good-humoured, elderly man, at times even handsome. He wore a suit of blue clothes, the skirts wide and old fashioned. He was the most trusted of all. I never saw any irregularity in his conduct, and once or twice I heard the servants say they looked to him to put down any disturbance in their absence. At times, however, he became agonized, and inflamed in the face, his features distorted, and he would lean forwards and thrust a handkerchief in his mouth, as if to stifle his feelings. It was then my spirits told me he was suffocating for me. He used to sit smoking, with his hands in his pockets, or play at cards, or read the papers. It was he that asked my pardon for assisting in the beginning to put me into the strait waistcoat: and when I was leaving the madhouse, he told me twice or thrice he should be ready to give evidence, if I called upon him as to my peculiar ill treatment; which he said had been very bad. He often used to joke good-humouredly with me, to show me kindness, and when under delusion I seized him to wrestle with him, he used to take it in sport, seize me by the collar, and shake me. He was a Roman Catholic; but they called him an infidel: as a Roman Catholic, he did not attend the chapel. I imagine he was a Deist.[145] He used to take away the Bible from me, saying, "you have read enough of it; it is that which brought you here." I thought it strange that the Lord Jehovah took away his own word from me: but my

---

145 Deists relied on reason rather than revelation to ground their ideas about God. From Perceval, not a compliment, but perhaps better than a Catholic.

spirits said, that since the redemption, all was changed, and that word was no longer necessary. I obeyed; but I did not understand. When I knelt to him as the Lord Jehovah, and to Herminet Herbert as Jesus Christ, in the evening, they would kneel before me in fun, which puzzled me extremely. Was this the goodness and condescension of the Lord? But my spirits told me the Lord took off my manner, and not the matter of my address. One day, on my calling him Jehovah, he replied with great promptitude, "Well! I *am* the Jehovah." I was constantly deluded to think that he, as my heavenly Father, would take me back to E———, where my family resided. Many absurdities did I attempt to perform in this hope. By ill luck he had resided in that neighbourhood when a boy, and knew all the lanes and houses about. He talked to me of lanes in which he had seen little groups of angels in the trees: this I was simple enough to believe; and all his remarks tended to confirm my deceptions.

One afternoon, I was left alone with him when yet fastened up; he brought three chairs, and lay down upon them, near me; holding in his hands a book or a paper from which he read. My spirits told me it was a delusion; that it was my fault if I did not mount to heavenly places, and see other things around me. They desired me to listen, and I heard two voices, one of Captain ———, reading the paper in a low voice to himself, another of a spirit from the same mouth, whispering things spiritual.

Mr. J. was the youngest patient in the room, and in my opinion the most cruelly treated. A young, gentlemanly, active, little man. I saw him occasionally naked in the bath, he was lightly and gracefully made. His hair was light, his face pale, his features plain; but at times his countenance was divine; at times, he looked dirty, sallow, mean, and loathsome. He used to talk a great deal and ask the other patients questions, or make remarks likely to offend, and impertinent, but, in my opinion, the utterance of a spirit of discernment or of divination. He used language figuratively, but I was not always able to understand his drift. He would ask, "have you brushed your coat this morning?" "will you let me brush your hat for you? are those shoes you have got on?" often he said to me, "do you fence?" I was so stupid as to take his questions simply at first; and I replied to him, that I had had lessons from Angelo; he then rejoined, "Angelo! aye, Angelo, they say Angelo fences well; for my part, I think he never had a foil in his hand in his life." Looking up into the sky once, he said to me, "do you see that beautiful woman?" He occasionally alluded to the doctrines of faith and good works; and I understood from him or others that he had belonged to a society of young men in Cambridge, who used language in a figurative manner, and held wild notions. I felt that he had meddled with matters too high for him. I need not say that no one appeared to comprehend him. Though all showed a dislike to his remarks, as if they knew they were being spoken *at* as well as spoken *to*. Hobbs used to act and look as if he suspected that there was a method in his madness; and I think Mr. Waldong knew as much, though he would not acknowledge it.

He often stood by me, when I was fastened up, and made allusions to my situation, asking me, Have you been at your father's house this morning? Do you make no efforts to get out from there, Mr. ———. Now the only thing I did besides singing aloud, hallooing (for which I got rated and trounced or flanked by the servant's duster) was to try and twist my neck, or to suffocate myself by pressing my nostrils against a small handle of wood fixed in the wall, which served as an arm to the seat in the niche. I imagined that he rebuked me, for not having yet executed my purpose, through cowardice and insincerity.

My spirits told me this was my youngest brother. I understood them literally at first, and I was perplexed because I could see but an imperfect resemblance in the features. But I was told that I did not like to see him; and therefore could not. Afterwards he was pointed out to me as my younger brother's Honesty; and I acknowledged a resemblance in character. He was allowed to remain with me alone upstairs, when I sat in the wicker chair after the opening of my temporal artery. One day, when I was at liberty, and the servants were gone out walking with most of the other patients, I sat at the table, after having attempted to play a game of drafts[146] with him, in which we did not succeed. I then began reading, and he sat down opposite to me, making observations on me aloud, which appeared to be condemnatory of me, and reflecting on my conduct. My spirits desired me to reply to them, or to leave the room. But I would not, and I contended against the spirits that called me out, if I remember, to defend my honour, obstinately resolved to do nothing till I was reduced to a state of the meanest and most debasing feelings I sat, through his remarks, in a spirit of malignity towards him for his impudence, and towards my Maker, resolved not to give up my position, for after being wearied and deluded by contradictory and unintelligible commands, I at times avenged myself by a complete revolt. A few days afterwards, whilst standing on the bank in the yard reading, I saw him coming out of the saloon, and walk down the alcove, his countenance was like that of Hyperion. He observed me, took displeasure at my demeanour, and halted,

---

146 Checkers.

making a remark. My spirits told me if I did not change my place or attitude, I should ruin his state of mind, and drive him to hell: for the love of God to change my place. I recollected the afternoon before mentioned, when he drove me to hell; and maintained my position, replying, that God who had insulted me through him, and had not protected me, might now protect him; in a few minutes he went down the yard—in appearance to me a devil.

He was often severely handled. He and Mr. J. the clergyman, were made to use the same indecent shower bath I was myself exposed to, I am afraid to say how long he was confined to the back-yard, without the privilege of exercise or of change of scene in accompanying us out walking: but I fear during the whole summer, he did not walk out so much as twenty-one days. A spirited, active, intelligent young man! I saw him once ask the servant to allow him to go out with tears in his eyes: but his hat was taken away from him, and the door locked in his face. Once he was not allowed to go out for ill conduct to myself, which Hobbs observed, for Hobbs often defended me from his impertinent intrusions. I would willingly have staid at home for him to go out, but I could not explain or express myself; and though his keen observations insulted me, I know he spoke to me the condemnation of a spirit in him, to which he was sincere, although I did not altogether understand him, for I had no time or place for reflection, or for self-examination; and my thoughts were too much confused. I was told his disorderly conduct prevented the keeper taking him out, and at the latter end of the year, when a powerful young lad whom I named Simplicity and Honesty, came to wait on us, there being then thirteen or fourteen patients in the room, I saw he was fastened to the lad's arm out walking, and struggling to get away from him. When left alone in the yard, he amused himself with picking up stones, climbing up into a small tree and sitting there looking over the country, and one day he picked nearly all the leaves off this tree.

I remember one day his shying small stones with great force in front of the lunatic's faces who were walking under the alcove; but I observed the stones never hit any one, and we were too near to be missed if he had meant us any harm. He cut at my legs with a knife under the table, but still to intimidate, not to do mischief, for he had opportunity to hurt me if he had designed it, before I changed my seat. I loved the young man, and one day by command of the spirits, I laid my head in his bosom, on the bench in the yard, but I could not understand the mind of the spirit in him. Towards the end of the year, I was provoked to strike him twice. One winter evening I was seated by the fire, reading a speech of my eldest brother, when my manner offended him who was sitting at the corner of the fire, on my right hand side. He asked me with a sneer "is that your speech or your brother's, sir," and on my making no reply, he alluded as the doctor had done once before, to my father's death. I was provoked to smite him over the lips with the pamphlet; he rose up sparring, and I rose and knocked him down. The servant coming in, and hearing the origin of the quarrel took my side; he went out of the room. I was applauded. The scene reminded me of passages in Roderick Random;[147] and I was full of grief.

Another evening in January, after I had been removed up stairs, and had been disputing with the doctor, and with my family, and had also received that treatment of my letters,

---

147 A satirical novel by Tobias Smollett following the adventures of a Scottish sailor.

and the replies, which exasperated me so much, and having had no exercise during the day, I went down to walk in the yard. Mr. J. took offence at me and shouldered me in passing two or three times. I took an attitude of preparation when he next came to me, he halted, and began sparring again; I was in no humour for sport, and fearing him, I struck him in the face, and gave him a bloody nose. His blood was very black. I am truly sorry for these blows, for I do not think now the young man designed to hurt me, but he was obeying a spirit of frolic and gaiety; on neither occasion did he offer to strike me again; but I could not command myself, being then desperate.

I have seen this young lad occasionally cleaning the shoes and knives in the knife hole, under the alcove; he always acted in a fitful manner, as if guided like myself by spiritual direction. When I began planning my escape, I observed him narrowly inspecting and considering the same points that I examined. When my spirits desired me to sing in the room, he stood by me and took up the air I began, or the song I was trying after, so as to help my memory. One day when I came home from walking, in the midst of the other gentlemen, I observed Mr. J. standing on the opposite side of the table at the further end. Hobbs passed behind me and along that side of the table, advancing towards him. I saw no violence or impropriety of conduct on his part, but in a minute a scuffle ensued between him and his keeper. During the whole of the struggle Mr. J. only exercised a passive resistance; determined, with great coolness to oppose and resist force, but not to exercise violence in return. He was dragged with extreme rudeness, resisting mightily, into the yard, and then down the alcove to a wooden seat, to which he was often manacled by the right wrist. I followed, desired by my spirits to take Mr. Fazakerley's position in the alcove as usual. The servant wanted to fasten Mr. J. on the seat by the manacle. Mr. J. resisted. The rascal got the young gentleman down on the bench, and whilst he vigorously, but still calmly, and only defensively struggled against him, seized him round the throat and strangled him. I was extremely excited, frightened, and grieved; for not having seen any cause for the attack upon the young man, indeed there had not been time for any, I more readily believed the voices that told me he was suffering for me, &c. And when I saw his bloated and inflamed cheeks, and the eyes starting out of the sockets, I offered to do any thing to rescue him. My spirits desired me to whirl myself round and round as fast as I could, which I did till I staggered against the wall, and nearly fell on the stone pavement. I attempted it a second time, being accused by my spirits of cowardice and insincerity; but either I really was afraid of a fall, or other sensations made me cease. The habitual submission of my spirit was such that I did not once think of attacking the servant. Now had I been in my sound senses I might have rushed on the man, seized him unawares, and dashed his head against the pavement. I speak as a man; for who can control his passion under every excitement, and what is nobler than to resent and punish cruel and brutal oppression? Then that which to a free man would have been counted an act of justifiable homicide in defence of a fellow creature, or at least but as an act of manslaughter, would have doomed me to perpetual banishment from society, as a madman, though an act noble in proportion to the danger that threatened me, whether I failed or succeeded. There are those in the world, I know, who will cruelly and coldly reply, that there was a difference, inasmuch as *the keeper was doing his duty*; and that at any rate to interfere in my case, would have proved my madness. These are the doctor's true friends. Vipers! I only hope I may catch them in the discharge of this *duty*, as I now am; and I will try to enlighten their consciences. When again I reflected on the brutal treatment which was attempted also on myself; I exclaimed, good God! but what must a man expect, even though not a surgeon, at the blood being thus forced up and coagulated in a lunatic's head. But with this shocking scene I must close my day's labour; painful, too painful at all times, but in this case, too much for me to reflect on patiently. God grant that I may not have undertaken this too late to do good to those I have left behind me!

Captain W. came into the common room in the summer time: when he first entered and peeped into the yard, he appeared to me as a son of Mr. Stuart Wortley's, a schoolfellow and a friend of my fourth brother; again he reentered from the yard, and I saw another of my schoolfellows, an Irishman and one of my friends. The likeness was so strong that I called out the names each time involuntarily. Mr. F. F. then introduced him to me as Captain W.; but having seen him before under the countenances of my friends, I did not believe him, but rather my spirits. He was a talkative young man of a religious mind, but slovenly. He told me that he had been obliged to leave his regiment on account of the state of his mind, and that his was a case of love madness. I said to him, if so, why not show more respect for his person, for the sake of his lady; he replied, oh! it did not signify here, in the world it signified, but what did it matter now? what were we sent here for? I thought it mattered here more than elsewhere, for he was not likely to get out unless he showed attention to his person. He was fully aware of his position.

He had come with his father, and had heard the arrangements made for him, which he detailed to me one day when complaining about pocket handkerchiefs not being supplied to him. I was entirely ignorant on what footing I was placed there. It was he that quizzed and terrified the simple old Quaker. He told me one day that he had attempted to make away with himself from the bars of a window upstairs: he used to talk of suicide openly, which was painful to hear. As I came gradually to my right mind, I used to burst into fits of laughter, at the discovery of the absurdity of my delusions, and of the still grosser absurdity of the conduct pursued towards me and the other patients; for at one time I could not control my humour, at another my anger; for I said, if it were only ridiculous, but now it is grossly cruel, selfish, and disgusting. Captain W. observing this, told me I should never get out of confinement, it was invariably observed that lunatics who laughed excessively, were incurable. I thought to myself, I'll not only get out, but laugh at you too into the bargain, good gentleman.

In the autumn, a respectable, silver haired, old clergyman, was added to our number. He was a tight, neat, busy, little man, and behaved, during the whole of his sojourn amongst us, with great decorum. He tried even to introduce the custom of saying grace at dinner, but it did not succeed. I saw no marks of insanity in him except at meals. The first time he sat down to dine with us, he refused his food, and in the presence of us all, for he was then sitting at the right side of the table, I was at the head of it; Hobbs seized him, and forced the victuals down his throat. It was a disgusting and frightful sight, to see the old man trembling, resisting, and to hear his suffocated sobs and cries. This scene was repeated several times at breakfast and dinner. At last the

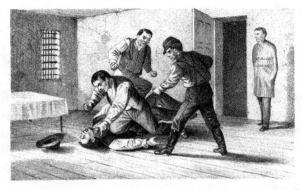

Ebenezer Haskell's narrative portrays the death of the patient Mr. Parks
as recounted by another patient at the Taunton Lunatic Asylum.

old gentleman was considered to be in his senses, and went
to church to give thanks for what was called his recovery,
before he went away. This patient talked to me sensibly and
rationally, he also worked with me in the shrubbery. One
afternoon in the yard, he began praising Dr. F.'s asylum, the
kindness, the humanity of the treatment. I replied, that I
begged leave to differ with him in toto. He asked me for
an example of conduct contrary to his opinions. I begged
his pardon if I wounded his feelings by mentioning his own
case; I asked if it was respectful to his age or to his profession, that he should have been so exposed before us, even if
it were necessary to force his food down his gullet; and if it
were considerate or humane to the spectators in any sense,
but more especially considering their state as lunatic and
nervous patients. He never spoke to me afterwards of the
humanity of the asylum.

In truth, the humanity of the asylum consisted in the
conduct of the patients, not in that of the system and of

its agents, for, had the patients felt or manifested half the indignation that nature or honour required of them, they would probably have been half murdered if not wholly so.

After the entrance of the Rev. Mr. ———, another Captain came in. He was a slovenly, imbecile, man, stooped very much, and laughed a great deal to himself. I understood that he had been removed from another asylum. I recollect nothing particularly of him, but that he flew out into very high words at tea one evening when I was left behind the other gentlemen gobbling my bread and butter, and mixing with it salt, pepper, and mustard, from a cupboard, in obedience to my spirits; he left the table saying, that he would not sit at it if I did not behave as a gentleman; I made no reply, but I was astonished at his interference; I felt, so long as the servants do not entertain the same opinion it matters very little to me here what you may think. I shall obey my spirits, do what you will with yours.

In the autumn, another elderly man was ushered one evening into the common room by one of the young doctors; it was immediately after the riots at Bristol. After a few words he was left alone. He was a decent, grey headed, short, hard featured, stubborn man, and appeared in every respect to be of sound mind. I imagined he was a gentleman who had come to visit one of the patients. My ideas were soon set right. It was towards tea time, and when he sat down at the table, he asked in a decided tone for some coffee; his request was at first met with silence; he repeated it, then Marshall, whom I called Sincerity, replied, "Oh! there is no coffee here, the tea is good enough for you." I thought, you have a severe lesson to learn, sir. The old man was of a very active body and mind. He had no employment, no one to converse with. At first he talked a great deal, with some wit; then he began to play tricks and was scouted; then his mind completely gave way: he used to go into the yard and daub himself with red soil calling it paint, and in a few weeks he was confined as I had been, in a straight waistcoat, upon the self-same seat, in the niche. His fall was rapid and shocking. One day before he was fastened up, whilst walking in the alcove, begrimed with dirt, and playing his pranks, Marshall ran behind him, and in joke, hit him a violent blow in the small of the back; the old man was put to great pain, for he said he had long had a complaint in the kidneys.

He was stiff in his joints from old age; when confined in the niche, he did not lose his spirits, but was still the noisiest and most talkative of us all; so that Captain W. asking us once which was the happiest man of us all, replied when all were silent, "old Mr. ———;" but I knew he was mistaken, and mistook spirits for happiness: the noise which men resort to, to hide themselves from themselves, and from one another, for real gaiety. He found out my name, and addressed me with a kind of forced and vulgar familiarity: he told me he was a merchant of the city of Bristol, and that one of his ancestors or relations had married a relation of my uncle, Sir John ———, whose family were of Somersetshire. He was a fine old man and I wondered at so much fun and enterprise in age, when youth seemed so supine.

He had originally been supercargo[148] in an East Indian ship, and had visited China. One day he showed me a privet leaf, saying it was a tea leaf, by which I understood his spirit meant it resembled, though he may have intended that it was, a tea leaf. He pretended to know a great deal, and to be able by skimming over a book, to acquire its contents. He

---

148   One who oversees the cargo on a merchant ship.

asked me to show him a pamphlet I was reading, in order to give a specimen of his talent; but he was not quiet; he did it to hide from others his own feelings, and to escape from his own ennui.

The treatment I had endured was shameful, but yet I was a young man. The treatment of this old man was horrible. All day long he was confined as I had been, on a wooden seat, amidst noise, insult, flippancy, and confusion. The common wants of nature were neglected in him. Oh! it was shocking. Of an evening, at his request, a request unheeded by Marshall the servant present, I held the box into which patients that smoke spate, for him as an urinal, emptying it afterwards in the yard. Often he was without even this decent aid. After sitting a whole day, in the evening I heard him begging for one of the hair cushions of the chairs, to put under him; no one attended to him; I did: the servant desired me not to do it, but I gave it to him. One Sunday young Mr. J. commenced flanking at his legs with a duster; I was so grieved that I put myself before him, to cover him, receiving the blows. I did not offer to strike Mr. J. for then I would not have lifted my hand voluntarily against any man, considering his body as the Lord's temple; but watching my opportunity, I snatched the duster away, gave it to Captain W. to keep, and went out of the room. The old man was grateful.

When I received and answered my letters, he used to ask me for pen and ink, pretending to write or direct a letter himself, but scrawling nonsense. He often inquired if there was no letter for him, and was disappointed and grieved in silence that there was none. He expected one from his child. I knew he would have to wait long. At last one came, and he received it eagerly.

One night I went up stairs to bed alone, and heard him call to me, for he slept in a room opening into the same passage: the servant not being yet with me, I went into his room. He was lying almost naked on the bed strapped down as I had been, but with a belt over his belly. He asked me I think for some water, which I gave him, and for other assistance which I was unable to render him; then I got to my own room not to be observed. He used to defile his bed night after night, for which the servants rated him, but I do not know that they struck him. Probably in behaving so he acted under a delusion, or nature gave way to necessity, having been controlled in the day time from delusion; perhaps also he was neglected.

On a Sunday evening, about three weeks after his entrance, when all were gone to church but Mr. Waldong and myself, he being very restless, I was surprised to see him get up, and collecting hastily chairs together, attempt to scale the alcove at the only feasible point for effecting an escape. Having formed as he thought his ladder he began changing his coat, to put on that of another. I said nothing but watched him, for he was putting in practice the scheme I had thought upon, and I thought if he succeeded I would be after him, if not, I was not suspected. One of the servants came in just as he was mounting.

Before I left the asylum, I was one day ordered to go down into the common room whilst Hobbs prepared to walk out with me, for then I used to walk out alone in a retired walk behind the kitchen garden. The room stank abominably; the rest of the gentlemen were in it, I inquired the cause, and I found it was owing to this old patient, who was seated at the end of the room tied up in his niche, not having had his bodily necessities attended to; yet he was left there an offence to himself and an insult to the other gen-tlemen. Once the same accident happened to myself, when the three humaner servants waited on us; but I was relieved from my situation as soon as they discovered it. I have sus-pected since that my dinner had been drugged.

I have already mentioned that I began writing to my family in November, to complain of the treatment which had been pursued towards me, and to find out to whom the blame was to be imputed. At the same time I demanded a private apartment, with a servant of my own choosing: that letter was opened and detained, in opposition to my wishes. I then wrote concisely to my eldest brother, that he might desire my letter to be given up to him, and insist upon my correspondence with my family being respected. The two letters were forwarded together. I was not sanguine in the expectation of obtaining my demand, I replied thus, if my family have been guilty of so great folly, as to submit me to such mismanagement, contrary to nature, reason, and reli-gion, there is no folly they may not be guilty of in respect of me: I was not surprised then as at a thing unexpected and impossible when my mother wrote to me word that she must be guided by the doctor as to my having a private apartment. I was still less surprised at a distinct refusal from *him*. Interest, prejudice, and pique, might influence his judgment; but I was astonished at the hardness of heart and want of understanding that could make an affectionate and indulgent parent doubt the reasonableness of my request; particularly when I knew that I was termed a nervous patient, and reflected that for years my mother had suffered from extreme nervousness, during which she could scarcely endure, and even forbade a newspaper being unfolded in her room; so greatly did she feel the need of quiet. Now I am sure that next to myself, no one will more acutely resent my illtreatment when she understands it, than my mother, and it is fearful to think how an habitual hardening the heart to misgivings of the mind respecting the trustworthiness of other men, and a supine surrender of the judgment, and of the dictates of honest feeling, to the impudent pretences of shallow hearted swindlers, may betray individuals, and whole classes, to the most shameful and inhuman acts of madness. Alas! it is too true, the treatment I have described can only be that of madmen or of villains. So opposite in nature to the end proposed!—I was not however able to brook my disappointment, it drove me almost mad through passion. Then it was that I struck the servant over the eye, and wrestled with others; then it was also I struck Mr. J.; then too, I foresaw and tried to prepare myself for all the difficulties and disappointments in the way of my obtaining my liberty with honour, resting my only hope on the enlightened character of the Lord High Chancellor, if by any means I might be able to gain his ear: I thank God he left me this hope, it buoyed me up though it proved partly false, my mind being blinded to the estimate I had long before made of men of public character, viz., that they are men great in one line, but devoid of real understanding; because, deciding wilfully, they reject light that restrains their activity, and contradicts their imperfect convictions.[149]

In consequence of my striking the servant a blow, I was desired to descend again, schoolboy fashion, into the common room, where I wrote with a sprained thumb as well as I could, my second appeal to my mother; in it I swore that

---

149 Perceval may have hoped that the Lord Chancellor would overturn his commitment to the asylum, or at least have allowed a "lunacy inquisition" in which Perceval could advocate on his own behalf.

I would have the life of one of the servants if I were not removed from that madhouse before three months were out. I could not patiently endure my situation, and it was indifferent to me if I was confined for life, so as I could avenge by blood the indignities I had been subjected to, and put an end to an agonizing state of suspense. If I were myself slain or hanged, death brought a joyful release, and no disgrace can I care for, having drunk the bitterest draughts of ill deserved ignominy, and despising as I do the accursed folly of the world. Fortunately I detailed in that letter a part of those indignities: my pride was wounded in so doing, for I could not brook that advantage was to be taken of my misfortunes to doubt my honour, but under the English lunatic doctors and the English country magistrates, I was obliged at last to have every feeling brutalized. My family had not, or pretended not to have been aware of my illtreatment. My mother desired by return of post that I might have a private room, and in a short time I had one. Then the ideas of all around me seemed to have changed towards me: my meals were private and served to me as to a gentleman, the familiarity of the servants seemed to cease, and to my broken spirit the exertions made to comply with my demands seemed excessive.

Fortunately there was a worthy and elderly physician residing in my mother's parish, who had formerly had the care of insane patients; she applied to him. He was a sensible, honest, humane man, but too mistrustful of his own sound judgment. He advised my mother to attend to my desires immediately, but on account of my violent language he could not look with calmness on my having a private lodging, or being with a private family. I learnt this from his own lips a year afterwards. I then demonstrated to him the extreme folly as well as cruelty of the conduct which had been pursued towards me even in this instance, and against which I had protested and remonstrated again and again without effect, viz., that resolutions were taken as to the disposal of my person and property, and communicated to me with about as much ceremony as if I were a piece of furniture, an image of wood, incapable of desire or will as well as of judgment. Steps were taken, but the reasons never shown to me, God knows it, never. My mother wrote to me to say that I was to be removed from the madhouse I was in, and to be confined in another; where, or under whom, was not mentioned, or why.[150] Had she mentioned her reasons for choosing another madhouse instead of a private lodging, I could have removed them immediately, and a long and painful altercation might have been prevented. I was not a madman acting with indiscriminate violence, but I was exasperated by the recollection of, and by actual suffering from insulting, degrading, cruel treatment. I had no ill-will to any individual, but to those concerned in the murder, the repeated murder of my spiritual and moral nature. On the contrary, I was in disposition like a child, in conduct, as I proved under these trying circumstances, calm and deliberative until rendered desperate. My resolution even to take the life of the keeper, though violent in expression, was determined in resolution and feeling, it was the cry of outraged human nature, not the victory of passion over right understanding. I still almost feel over again what I then felt.

So little care was taken by my relations to be precise or explanatory in their conduct towards me, that the

---

150   Upon leaving Dr. Fox's asylum in Brislington, Perceval would be placed in Ticehurst Asylum under the care of Dr. Charles Newington. He would write about this experience at length in the 1840 edition of his text.

previous letter I received from my mother, desiring me a private apartment, merely contained a refusal to remove me from the madhouse of Dr. F.: the next told me that a private apartment was being prepared for me in a madhouse elsewhere. By that time I had been again insulted and injured by the forced use of the shower bath and cold bath. I considered my life in danger under insolent and violent servants, malignant, prejudiced, and nettled physicians. The magistrates called, and I claimed their interference: I stated that I was much grieved to be compelled to appeal to them against my mother, but that her conduct was so unjust that I was afraid I must look to them for legal assistance if she did not answer my letter according to my reasonable desires. They in a loose way promised me the assistance of a lawyer, but had I needed one they left me the name of no party to whom I could apply, and I must have waited three months to make my next appeal. So the convalescent madman who needs most help, is left most of all to his own resources; and the doctors have ample time to drive him insane again, or to provoke him to acts of indiscretion, that may be construed into proofs of derangement.[151]

I now took up this attitude against my family. I argued that although I was unsettled in my judgment and still partially lunatic, it did not give mankind or them any legal right to exercise a brutal and tyrannical control over my will, without respect to the nature of my calamity, and to the degree of restoration I had attained to. Instead of being treated as I was, *de haut en bas*,[152] with complete contumely,

---

151 These sentiments would be among the most influential in Perceval's later advocacy work—namely, the difficulty facing an incarcerated person who has recovered from their illness and is unable to effect their freedom, and the failures of the current inspection system.

152 French: from height to lowness, that is, condescendingly.

no argument or address being made to my understanding, I
conceived that my being a lunatic required on the contrary
the more scrupulousness on their part, the more caution,
openness, and explanation. That it was their duty to make
my way more straight and clear before me because I was by
my disease already sufficiently prone to delusion, and even
to unprovoked suspicion. So at least the doctors desire you
to believe, but I question if the suspicions of lunatics are not
often most sane, and engendered necessarily by the under-
hand dealings of others towards them. There is a distinction
to be made between the suspicions of lunatics and that of
lunacy. I considered that though surrendered by law to the
charge of a physician, it was to be protected, and to be prevented from injuring others, not to lay me open helpless and
defenceless to his villanies, and his treachery; to the violence
of his servants, or to experiments of his quackery upon my
constitution and feelings under the pretence of cure, and
that even if it were so, the law could not justify him in a
system brutally perverse and contrary to all science, surgical
or moral; a system unnatural and impudent; that the silence
of the law could not be an excuse for it, if no patient had
hitherto had understanding or courage to plead against it. I
determined therefore for safety, for example's sake, and for
revenge to appeal to the law against my physician. I avowed
the three motives.

In order to succeed I desired first legal assistance to set
forth my case and to save my rights; secondly to be taken
to London to be for a short time under the care of a surgeon who had known me from a child, that he witnessing
my state of mind and body, and hearing my complaints,
might be able to argue and to give evidence concerning
the necessity of requiring me to use the cold bath, at that

inclement season, the propriety of using force considering the degree of understanding I was restored to, and the danger to my health of body from the shock and cold, and to my mind from the needless excitement. These requests were denied.[153] I then wrote to my mother, stating to her, that if she really was not aware of the cruelty of my situation, she had been deceived by Dr. F., and then might justly join me in demanding legal satisfaction, but that if she did not do so, I could not be reconciled to her, and must hold her also responsible to me at law, for she was certainly the most culpable. Moreover, that though I knew I was still lunatic, yet I knew too, from sad experience, that I was capable of taking care of myself in a more reasonable manner than the wretched physicians she confided in; that I was not a lunatic incapable of controlling myself, although I felt so sensible of my need of observation that I would not accept my liberty if it were given to me, but should place myself immediately under the eye of some one I could rely upon; but that if she insisted on placing me, where under pretence of observation, I should be defenceless, open to violence, impertinent intrusion, indelicate treatment, and deprived of tranquillity, peace, rest, and security, I should claim my freedom, though lunatic, as one not mischievous, and hold her responsible for my future detention.

In taking this resolution I was actuated also by the desire of convincing the consciences of my mother and of my family, to see the sin they had been guilty of. Knowing the terrors of the Lord, knowing what it was of horror to feel that repentance comes too late, I stood in awe of God

---

153   In Perceval's 1840 edition, he will write at length about his requests to visit doctors of his own choosing as soon as possible after leaving Dr. Fox's asylum in order to obtain evidence of his abuse. The doctor at his new asylum rejected this request repeatedly.

if I did not rebuke them, and shocked at their doom if they should die unconvinced and hardened against my rebuke: for I call God to witness, although accused by my family at the instigation of the doctors of lunacy as if devoid of affection, I endured continual and deep agony of mind, affection and attachment, contending within me with feelings of duty and just wrath. The conduct I endured was not to be endured in life with patience: the stupidity of spiritual death alone submits to it quietly. The judgment that I came to, that it was my duty to sacrifice affection and attachment to the maintenance of my rights, and to rescue myself and others from treatment revolting to humanity, to enlighten the minds of others by bringing down condemnation on the guilty, even though that guilty one was my ———. I cannot write the word; and this, under the charge of being cruel and unnatural, to save the soul: this judgment may have been mistaken, but it was not that of a madman, and no man can rebuke me for it who has not passed through like extremities.

I might as well have appealed to the winds. I received letters from my elder brother and his wife, canting about submission, patience, and the Holy Spirit; to which I replied in mockery and disdain. I knew that my patience had been proved in a fire they could not have stood under for a moment; that it had not given way until they had neglected my representations, and made me desperate; and they talked to me of patience, ignorant of facts and circumstances, whose business it was to have humbled themselves and to have applied patiently for information to me. *They* wrote to me of the Holy Ghost by *whose* conduct I was driven well nigh, and at last altogether to blaspheme the holy name of God, and to doubt his Providence. *They* talked to me of my Heavenly Father's will, *who* if they had allowed their stubborn stupidity, and hypocritical reliance on the doctor to have been pierced by one cry of agony, ought to have known that they were already guilty before my Heavenly Father of that perverse will by which I was abandoned, through which I was destroyed, and wander about the ruin of what I was, and to which I was still compelled to address threats, argument, and representation. Another wrote to me actually defending the doctor in opening my letters, taking the part of my enemy, and reasoning against me. I was so disgusted at his indelicacy and presumption, for he always wrote to me as if *he* knew what lunacy was, not I who had endured it, therein proving the stubborn and innate lunacy of human nature, rushing to give an opinion where nothing is known to found a right opinion upon; that I wrote on the note a few laconic lines to say, that I returned him his note, and that until he changed his mind and expressed his sorrow to me for having written it, I could not have any communion of spirit with him, and therefore desired not to speak with him.

When indeed I desired my correspondence to be respected, it was from feelings of delicacy towards my family, as much as to myself. But I met with no delicacy in return. I wonder at their insensibility, how that intelligent and sensitive souls can become so besotted. But I am wrong, human nature has yielded to the absurd and immodest assumptions of the papal church in regard of confession; there are other vipers as subtle. But others behaved in like manner. When I made my first appeal to the magistrates, in doing which, confined in a madhouse, recovering from lunacy, weakened by long sickness, I had to conciliate resentment and exasperation, with respect and filial duty, vindictive feelings, with affection; I had to speak in presence of nine or ten magistrates, servants, and doctors. None had the delicacy to withdraw, no one had the gentlemanly feeling to desire me to see them in private. They stared with impudent and unmeaning curiosity. Nay, I have one exception to make. Captain W., confined like me as a lunatic, left the room; he afterwards apologized to me for being in it, saying, he was unaware of what I was going to speak about, but that the moment he heard me he retired. I thanked him, and told him, that I should have been glad, amongst so many unfeeling, stupid, and suspicious judges, to have had one honest, clever, and gentlemanly witness to my complaints and demeanour.

At last the letter came to announce my mother's determination to remove me from that madhouse to another. I wrote immediately objecting to my person being bandied about across the country at the discretion of others, I knew not whither, without the slightest respect to my inclination or judgment. I demanded again a private lodging and a servant of my own choosing,*[154] by which I meant, that I should have a voice in his appointment, and continuing with me, the only true safeguard against disrespectful conduct. I refused to accede to her desires; I held her responsible for my detention; and I desired that I might be placed in a neighbourhood where my name was known, and my personal character might be respected by the magistrates. I repeated my request to be brought to town if only for three weeks to see the surgeon alluded to above, and to take the advice of a lawyer; also to have my teeth attended to, which were in a state of decay, not having been washed for a whole year. I

---

154 [Perceval's note] *This expression was unfortunately mistaken, as if I wanted to have a servant of my own instead of selecting one of the doctor's; for this reason it was refused; but the reason was not communicated to me, or I might have explained it, instead of being condemned without knowing it, as absurd.*

also prayed that whithersoever my journey, I might not be compelled to travel more than six hours a day: for I feared that fatigue and excitement might overcome me, my nerves being so shattered, my frame so weak. Learning afterwards that my elder brother was to remove me, I wrote a letter to him, rebuking him for his conduct to me, for his neglect of my letters, and inattention to my requests; I refused also my hand to him, and to speak to him unless he acknowledged his fault, and asked my pardon: I consider it my duty to deal truly by them, and I was obliged to act concisely, because I was often deprived of the power of speech, and could not trust to myself to moderate my expressions, or to them to respect me if I spoke in a broken, irregular manner. My spirits often counselled me to disguise all my resentment until I was clear of Dr. F.'s establishment. It might have been better for me: but then I replied, "I must play the hypocrite, which I cannot do long," and my mind shrunk at the idea of deceiving my own relations with a design to punish them, besides, I was not able to endure the treatment I received any longer, therefore I chose the straightforward path.

When they arrived, I returned to my other brother, as I intended, the note he had written. I was amused, perplexed, and provoked at the same time by the familiarity of their demeanour towards me, in spite of my reserve. I understood my position immediately, and saw my little hope, and the great difficulties before me: that I had no chance of success so long as I argued with my relations alone. For why? they looked on me as a misguided child; but I despised them as dupes of their own conceit, and guilty of grosser lunacy and insanity in their dealings towards me without the excuse of derangement, than I had been the victim of in my trouble. A wise man can hardly accept or admit the rebuke of a wise man; how much less could my infatuated brothers admit the justice of the rebuke of one whom they condemned as luna-tic without discrimination.

To check the misplaced familiarity of my elder brother, I asked him if he had received no letter from me, he said, yes, and I resumed my silence; but I think when we halted for the night, I found he alluded to a letter of a previous date. He then told me he had received no other, but that Dr. F. had just put into his hands two or three letters which he had as usual opened and detained. Alas! if these letters had been sent they might have changed my mother's mind, and saved her and my family from two years of wretched con-tention with me, and exposure, and myself from two years' cruel and unjust confinement. They as well as I reaped the bitter fruits of surrendering their judgments to the prepos-terous and impudent claims to confidence of ignorant and charlatan practitioners; and of neglecting the complaints of a lunatic relation, restored at that time to a purer and truer sense of religion and propriety than they possessed, although not correct in all his understanding.

For by what right can a doctor presume to pry into the secrets of a patient's conscience, who is not only a per-fect stranger to him, but also a gentleman—to overlook the affections and the desires of his heart? and what right have his relations to presume on their authority to betray a patient's and a gentleman's feelings into such hands? They confess themselves ignorant of the nature of the disease they handle; they show themselves wilfully so, and it stands to reason that as far as the mind and morals are concerned, they cannot pretend to so much fitness as the relations of the lunatic; moving as mine do in a higher class, educated to finer feelings and to use much more consideration. They neglect their duties even as surgeons or as physicians; the dictates of common sense they make light of; let them mind their own duties at least, before they trespass beyond their line. But their impudent presumption is beyond calculation. If any particular kindness had been shown to me, if any persuasion, exhortation, or investigation, had been diligently used towards me, then to pry into my secret griefs or follies, might have been excusable; the zeal, however misplaced, was consistent. But ruined in body and in mind, I was left to help myself out of the dilemma as I could, and what is more, surrounded with every difficulty. When too, in spite of their cruelty and exposure of me, my constitution triumphed over riot and severity, where peace and indulgence were required; and my mind by its own efforts, shook off the appalling chains of delusion: these wise, clever, at least cunning men, heaped every obstacle in my way to health, in my return to sound society. Climbing out of the well into which they had thrown me, the stones fell down upon me, wounding and crushing me in my advance, or hurling me again to the bottom.

The clergymen of the established church ought to have the superintendence of the mental wants and infirmities of the deranged members of their communion, and the two offices of physician to the body and physician to the soul, distinct in nature, should be equally respected.[155] Sovereigns in this country, their ministers, and the people have been guilty of a great crime in neglecting this important distinction, and the hierarchy have betrayed their office. Yet who can wonder at that who knows how they are appointed? A

---

155   This idea would remain a principle of Perceval's advocacy, but others in the Alleged Lunatics' Friend Society were uncomfortable with religious involvement in civil matters. His rejection of the practice of reading patients' mail would also be a common refrain.

respectable clergyman, however, unless he were entitled by the ties of friendship or of affection, would not presume to do by treachery or by compulsion, that which these men do without any title; and in spite of the remonstrances of their patients. There can be only one excuse for a doctor opening the letters of his patients, and that is when the patient is without friends and without relations who take any interest in him. It is obvious, however, that it is unjust that the doctor should at any time have a summary control over the patient's correspondence, and where a patient has connexions, that in many respects, interference in the privacy of that correspondence may be improper; whatever mystery may hang over the origin of the disorder of any individual, whatever absurdities or worse than absurdities he may write, his relations are the most worthy to be first trusted with that mystery, and they ought to shield those absurdities and irregularities from the ridicule and from the officious scrutiny of strangers. They ought to judge after inspection, what parts of the correspondence may be communicated to the physician, and this not without self-respect and the respect due to the character and to the misfortunes of one who cannot control his feelings, and who exposes the nakedness of his heart, in a state of exasperation and of delusion.

When I left the doctor's parlour for the last time I bowed to the old man and Mr. F. F. without speaking. I shook hands with the other son, he was not to blame, and had shown me kindness. The eldest of the two maliciously replied; "Good bye, Mr. ———, I wish I could give you hopes of your recovery." A vile and cold speech towards me, and as it regarded my two unfortunate brothers: but they deserved it. My relations with Dr. F. were compulsory. Thank God I knew that I was recovering, and knew their hollowheartedness;

therefore I was more shocked at the possibility of such expressions being used to a patient who might not be able to endure them, than I was myself discouraged, or disinclined to act upon the judgment I had formed of their conduct and of their principles.

SOLI DEO GLORIA.[156]

THE END.

---

156   Latin: Glory to God alone.

Note.—The Letters promised in an appendix at the end of the volume have been suppressed on the ground of delicacy by the advice of my Publisher.

J. HADDON, CASTLE STREET, FINSBURY.[157]

---

157   Finsbury is in London.

ACKNOWLEDGMENTS

I WOULD LIKE TO THANK Will Fenton, one-time Director of Research and Public Programs at the Library Company of Philadelphia, for the invitation to edit this volume, and Rachel D'Agnostino, Curator of Printed Books, for her time and expertise as she created a manuscript of Perceval's text based on the Library Company's edition and digitized images for inclusion.

Enormous thanks also to the staff at Lanternfish Press for envisioning this project and including me in it. Thanks to Christine Neulieb for conversation about Perceval's errant commas and her keen edits of my own, to Amanda Thomas for producing the volume, and to Feliza Casano for demystifying the mystical marketing process.

Thanks to Sander Gilman for his support and for lending his ear and eye to this project.

Finally, I write with gratitude for John Perceval, who shared his story, and for the others who have done the same. I wish that more people had the chance.

SOURCES

Bateson, Gregory, ed. *Perceval's Narrative: A Patient's Account of His Psychosis, 1830-1832*. New York: William Morrow & Company, 1974.

Encyclopaedia Britannica. Chicago: Encyclopædia Britannica, 2021. www.britannica.com.

Fox, Francis and Charles Fox. *History and Present State of Brislington House near Bristol, an Asylum for the Cure and Reception of Insane Persons*. Bristol: Light and Ridler, 1836.

Funk & Wagnalls New World Encyclopedia. Chicago: World Almanac Education Group, Inc., 2020. EBSCOhost.

Hervey, Nicholas. "Advocacy or Folly: The Alleged Lunatics' Friend Society, 1845-63." *Medical History* 30 (1986): 245-275.

Hickman, Clare. "The Picturesque at Brislington House, Bristol: The Role of Landscape in Relation to the Treatment of Mental Illness in the Early Nineteenth-Century Asylum." *Garden History* 33, no. 1 (2005): 47-60.

Hunter, Richard and Ida Macalpine. "John Thomas Perceval (1803-1876) Patient and Reformer." *Medical History* 6, no. 4 (1962): 391-95.

Marcel, Michael. "The Tongues Revival 1830." Accessed November 19, 2021. https://ukwells.org/revivalists/the-tongues-revival-1830#

McCandless, Peter. "Liberty and Lunacy: The Victorians and Wrongful Confinement." In *The Social History of Psychiatry in the Victorian Era*, edited by Andrew Scull, 339-362. Philadelphia: University of Pennsylvania Press, 1981.

Oxford Dictionary of National Biography. Oxford: Oxford University Press, 2021. www.oxforddnb.com

Oxford English Dictionary. Oxford: Oxford University Press, 2021. www.oed.com.

[Perceval, John.] *A narrative of the treatment experienced by a gentleman, during a state of mental derangement; designed to explain the causes and the nature of insanity, and to expose the injudicious conduct pursued towards many unfortunate sufferers under that Calamity*. London: Effingham Wilson, 1838.

Perceval, John. *A narrative of the treatment experienced by a gentleman, during a state of mental derangement; designed to explain the causes and the nature of insanity, and to expose the injudicious conduct pursued towards many unfortunate sufferers under that Calamity.* London: Effingham Wilson, 1840.

Perceval, John. "Treatment of the Insane." *Provincial Medical and Surgical Journal* 15, no. 24 (1851): 665-666.

Report from the Select Committee on Lunatics; Together with the Proceedings of the Committee, Minutes of Evidence, Appendix, and Index. Printed for the House of Commons, 1859.

"Revolting riots in Queen Square." *BBC Bristol*, April 27, 2004, https://www.bbc.co.uk/bristol/content/madeinbristol/2004/04/riot/riot.shtml.

Shorter, Edward. *A History of Psychiatry: From the Era of the Asylum to the Age of Prozac.* New York: Wiley, 1997.

Smith, Leonard. "A Gentleman's Mad-Doctor in Georgian England: Edward Long Fox and Brislington House." *History of Psychiatry* 19, no. 2 (2008): 163-184.

Wise, Sarah. *Inconvenient People: Lunacy, Liberty, and the Mad-Doctors in Victorian England.* Berkeley: Counterpoint, 2012.

ILLUSTRATIONS

Esquirol, Etienne. *Des maladies mentales considérées sous les rapports médical, hygiénique et médico-légal.* Paris: Chez J.-B. Baillière, Libraire de l'acadèmie royale de médecine, Rue de L'École-de-médecine, N. 17.; Londres: Même Maison, 219, Regent Street.; Lyon: Chez Ch. Savy.; Leipsig: Chez L. Michelsen., 1838. Courtesy of the Library Company of Philadelphia: 112172.O (Rosenberg).

Fox, Francis Ker. *History and present state of Brislington House near Bristol: an asylum for the cure & reception of insane persons, established by Edward Long Fox MD. A:D. 1804 and now conducted by Francis & Charles Fox MD.D.* Bristol: Light & Ridler, 1836. Courtesy of the Wellcome Collection.

Haskell, Ebenezer. *The trial of Ebenezer Haskell, in lunacy, and his acquittal before Judge Brewster, in November, 1868: together with a brief sketch of the mode of treatment of lunatics in different asylums in this country and in England, with illustrations, including a copy of Hogarth's celebrated painting of a scene in Old Bedlam, in London, 1635.* Philadelphia: E. Haskell, 1869. Courtesy of the Library Company of Philadelphia: 18389.O.

Swan, Moses. *Ten years and ten months in lunatic asylums in different states.* Hoosick Falls [N.Y.]: Printed for the author, 1874. Courtesy of the Library Company of Philadelphia: 114188.D (Rosenberg).

Workman, Juliet. *The cornets: or The hypocrisy of the Sisters of Charity unveiled.* Baltimore: John W. Woods, 1877. Courtesy of the Library Company of Philadelphia: 114262.D (Rosenberg).

FURTHER READING

Agnew, Anna. *From Under the Cloud; or, Personal Reminiscences of Insanity.* Cincinnati: Robert Clarke: 1886.

Ben-Moshe, Liat. *Decarcerating Disability: Deinstitutionalization and Prison Abolition.* Minneapolis: University of Minnesota Press, 2020.

Ben-Moshe, Liat, Chris Chapman, and Allison C. Carey, eds. *Disability Incarcerated: Imprisonment and Disability in the United States and Canada.* New York: Palgrave Macmillan, 2014.

Bly, Nellie. *Ten Days in a Mad-House.* New York: Ian L. Monro, 1877.

Bulwer Lytton, Rosina. *A Blighted Life.* London: The London Publishing Office, 1880.

Burch, Susan. *Committed: Remembering Native Kinship in and beyond Institutions.* Chapel Hill: University of North Carolina Press, 2021.

Collins, Wilkie. *The Woman in White.* London: Penguin Classics, 1999 [1860].

Denny, Lydia. *Statement of Mrs. Lydia B. Denny, Wife of Reuben S. Denny, of Boston, in Regard to Her Alleged Insanity.* Boston: 1862.

Dully, Howard and Charles Fleming. *My Lobotomy: A Memoir.* New York: Three Rivers Press, 2008.

Foucault, Michel. *Madness and Civilization: A History of Insanity in the Age of Reason.* Translated by Richard Howard. New York: Vintage, 1988.

Geller, Jeffrey and Maxine Harris, eds. *Women of the Asylum: Voices from Behind the Walls, 1840-1945.* New York: Anchor Books, 1994.

Gilman, Sander. *Seeing the Insane: A Visual and Cultural History of Our Attitudes Toward the Mentally Ill.* Brattleboro: Echo Point Books & Media, 2014.

LeFrançois, Brenda, Robert Menzies, and Geoffrey Reaume. *Mad Matters: A Critical Reader in Canadian Mad Studies.* Toronto: Canadian Scholars' Press Inc., 2013.

Metzl, Jonathan. *The Protest Psychosis: How Schizophrenia Became a Black Disease.* Boston: Beacon Press, 2011.

Paternoster, Richard. *The Madhouse System.* London: George Stuart, 1841.

Penney, Darby and Peter Stastny. *The Lives They Left Behind: Suitcases from a State Hospital Attic.* New York: Bellevue Literary Press, 2009.

Peterson, Dale, ed. *A Mad People's History of Madness.* Pittsburgh: University of Pittsburgh Press, 1982.

Reiss, Benjamin. *Theaters of Madness: Insane Asylums and Nineteenth-Century American Culture.* Chicago: University of Chicago Press, 2008.

Scull, Andrew. *Madness in Civilization: A Cultural History of Insanity from the Bible to Freud , from the Madhouse to Modern Medicine.* Princeton: Princeton University Press, 2016.

Showalter, Elaine. *The Female Malady: Women, Madness and English Culture, 1830-1980.* London: Virago Press, 1985.

Stone, Elizabeth. *Exposing the Modern Secret Way of Persecuting Christians in Order to Hush the Boice of Truth. Insane Hospitals are Inquisition Houses. All Heaven is Interested in This Crime.* Boston: 1859.

Summers, Martin. *Madness in the City of Magnificent Intentions: A History of Race and Mental Illness in the Nation's Capital.* Oxford: Oxford University Press, 2019.

Szasz, Thomas, ed. *The Age of Madness.* Garden City, NY: Anchor Books, 1973.

Wise, Sarah. *Inconvenient People: Lunacy, Liberty, and the Mad-Doctors in Victorian England.* Berkeley: Counterpoint, 2012.

Wong, Alice, ed. *Disability Visibility: First-Person Stories from the Twenty-First Century.* New York: Vintage, 2020

ABOUT THE EDITOR

LINDSEY GRUBBS is faculty in the Department of Public Health at California State University, East Bay, where she teaches courses in ethics and humanities. With a doctorate in English and postdoctoral training in bioethics, she researches the cultural history and contemporary ethics of psychiatry and neuroscience.

YOU MIGHT ALSO ENJOY...

CLOCKWORK EDITIONS
Carmilla
by Joseph Sheridan LeFanu
edited by Carmen Maria Machado

*Medusa's Daughters: Magic and Monstronsity
from Women Writers of the Fin-de-Siècle*
edited by Theodora Goss

The King in Yellow
by Robert W. Chambers
edited by John Edgar Browning

FICTION
The Quelling
by Barbara Barrow

The City of Folding Faces
by Jayinee Basu

*The Vampire Gideon's Suicide Hotline &
Halfway House for Orphaned Girls*
by Andrew Katz